SUPER SIMPLE INTERMITTENT FASTING FOR WOMEN OVER 70

Reignite your Metabolism, Achieve Weight Loss, and Embrace Ageless Living

Mattie B. Rivera

TABLE OF CONTENTS

INTRODUCTION

Welcome aboard to an exciting journey that could be the most invigorating decision you will take this year! As a seasoned nutritionist, I'm eager to introduce you to the life-changing benefits of intermittent fasting, especially designed for the dynamic women who are 70 and beyond. You are the embodiment of wisdom and strength, and it's your time to flourish in this season of your life.

Growing older is a natural process, but that doesn't mean you have to accept a decline in your health. Now's the moment to steer your wellness in a new direction, one that promises to refresh your physical, mental, and emotional well-being. I admit, I was once skeptical about intermittent fasting, dismissing it as a passing trend. However, it's been a game-changer for me, and I'm excited to pass on this freedom to you.

We, as women past 70, encounter distinct challenges. Hormonal shifts can interfere with adopting new routines, and there's a common misconception that our prime days are long gone. I'm here to debunk that myth! With proper guidance and encouragement, you can defy those myths and experience renewed energy.

After diving deep into research, chatting with healthcare experts, and drawing from my own journey, I've put together a detailed guide tailored for women's unique requirements at this stage in life. Get ready to uncover the amazing perks of intermittent fasting, including sharper thinking, a boost in vitality, and better control over your weight.

But this book offers more than a fasting regimen – it's an integrated approach to living well. Inside, you'll find actionable advice for reducing stress, improving sleep, and indulging in self-care, all customized for you. Tasty recipes, structured meal plans, and list of handy mobile apps that can facilitate your success.

So, let's embark on this transformative path together. Harness the power of intermittent fasting and begin a new chapter brimming with health, confidence, and delight. You've got this, and I'm thrilled to walk with you every step of the way!

CHAPTER ONE

THE EVOLUTION OF INTERMITTENT FASTING: FROM ANCIENT RITUALS TO MODERN HEALTH TREND

The current trend sees intermittent fasting as the most contemporary form of fasting. It has advanced in time and is mainly employed for health objectives and weight reduction. In simple terms, intermittent fasting means you follow a specific eating routine that involves alternating periods of not eating (fasting) and regular food intake.

Intermittent fasting is not something brand new. It has existed for many centuries and people from different cultures and religions across the globe have been practicing it for a long time. In the past, people fasted for various reasons; it could be religious, medical, or because there was not enough food available.

Fasting, an old method of healing, has its roots in history. Numerous cultures have revered it over time but the Greeks, with their dedication to medicine and philosophy appreciated this practice greatly. A well-known doctor from Greece named Hippocrates believed that fasting might assist sick individuals. He suggested that sometimes not eating or drinking could help the body heal. According to Hippocrates, fasting is not only about not eating food. It's also a method to let your body clean itself, improve how you feel and think clearer. He considered it helpful for the body's self-healing process.

Plato and Aristotle, two famous Greeks, believed fasting was beneficial too. Plato spoke of how it would aid individuals in managing their wants and enhance their capacity for thought. Similarly, Aristotle - who possessed extensive knowledge across numerous fields - opined that moderation in food consumption was vital to maintain good condition of both body and intellect.

Fasting is also a part of several religions (like Islam, Christianity, and Buddhism). It helps in purifying or cleansing the soul and gaining spiritual benefits such as getting nearer to God. These religious customs are still observed by many people worldwide even in present times. During the mid-1800s, E.H. Dewey made known in his book "The True

Science of Living "that the majority of illnesses are dietary. This began a trend of long-term fasting. In medical literature, there are early documented cases of people fasting for 30-40 days which happened between 1880 and 1890.

Around 1900, investigation into how fasting affects obesity started to become more significant. The Fasting Cure, a book written by Upton Sinclair in 1911, brought fasting and its possible health advantages into greater public focus.

Folin and Denis in 1915 proposed that many short periods of starvation should be used to decrease weight, while long-term sessions would be reserved for extreme obesity situations. In the year 1945, they started to experiment with intermittent fasting on lab rats.

From the start of the 20th century, research was initiated by scientists to understand the possible health advantages of fasting. One of these early investigators is Dr. Luigi Cornaro, an Italian nobleman who existed during the 15th century and wrote a book named "The Art of Living Long" promoting a diet that included fasting periods (n.d.).

Now, let's move ahead to the 21st century where intermittent fasting is a trendy topic for health. In the last two decades, there has been a consistent rise in interest in intermittent fasting. This can be attributed to numerous scientific studies focusing on animals and humans alike, along with an expanding attention from media sources.

Intermittent fasting is gaining popularity because it's not difficult to do. You don't need to go through many days of extreme hunger to experience a wide range of mental and physical improvements. The public attention to intermittent fasting's is also connected to its promotion by celebrities and the spread of before-and-after images on social media platforms. To sum up, intermittent fasting has been around for ages, from ancient traditions to today's health fads. It's been praised by famous figures like Hippocrates, Plato, and Aristotle for its health benefits.

As we proceed, we will take a closer look at how intermittent fasting might help our health and what risks it might pose. We'll explore how it affects things like weight, thinking ability, and overall health. But we'll also talk about who might need to be careful with fasting, especially if they have health issues or follow special diets.

UNLOCKING THE FOUNTAIN OF YOUTH: THE UNEXPECTED BENEFITS OF INTERMITTENT FASTING FOR WOMEN OVER 70

A lady who has seen many sunrises may be seasoned, but it does not imply she is ready to disappear. By society's measure, crossing sixty-five categorizes you as a senior. However, these numbers cannot truly express the feelings of a woman. The body might age at its own speed but usually, the mind remains lively. It is often the reflection in the mirror that reminds us we are not as youthful as before.

As people grow older, their focus switches from outer looks to inner health. Yet a study has shown that even though many aged, ladies say they want to lose weight for better health, the main reason often ends up being plain old vanity. Many years have passed, but still, some women desire a weight that makes them feel attractive and confident.

Intermittent fasting is one method that can assist elderly people to appear and feel healthier. It's not only about losing weight; it may also enhance energy levels while promoting longevity. The main good effect of intermittent fasting is its support for autophagy, a process in cells that helps to take out damaged cells and initiate repair. To grasp the reason why this style of fasting is seen as a powerful anti-aging instrument, it is necessary to depict what this process exactly involves:

Events That Occur After Food Consumption

Every organ in our body (heart, brain, liver, and muscles) requires energy to work. We obtain this energy from the food we consume. The food we eat gets mixed within our bodies using fluids (acid and enzymes) found in the stomach, for digestion. The carbohydrates (sugar and starches) from this food are changed into glucose - a kind of sugar.

The stomach and intestinal walls, take in the glucose and then let it go into blood. Glucose goes through the bloodstream to different organs where it acts as their main energy supply. The glucose can be used right away for power or kept in our bodies, ready to be used later. The extra glucose is either saved as glycogen in the liver, smooth muscle cells, adipose tissue (even small amounts in brain and blood cells!) or turned into fat.

Events that Occur When Fasting

During the period between meals, when the body is in a fasted state, the liver changes glycogen into glucose for continuous energy supply. On an average note, a person who does not engage in such activity will use up their glycogen stores within 10-12 hours. But for someone who exercises, this process happens more quickly since the body requires extra energy while doing physical activities.

After the liver's glycogen reserve is finished, the body starts using energy from adipose tissue (body fat). This fat can be found in many places throughout our body: under our skin (known as subcutaneous fat), around organs inside us like the heart and liver area (referred to as visceral or "belly" fats), among muscles, within the bone marrow and even in breast tissue.

In the situation of the body using energy stored in adipose tissue, fats are divided into free fatty acids. These acids convert into more metabolic fuel in the liver. So, when fasted condition continues for a certain duration, the body burns fat to produce energy and reduces its extra fat content.

Cell Growth in the Well-fed States

When you are not hungry, the cells in your body are in a state where they grow. Insulin signaling and mammalian target of rapamycin (mTOR) pathways, which tell cells to divide and make new proteins that provoke growth, get stimulated when you eat enough food.

When there are many nutrients, particularly carbohydrates and proteins, the mTOR pathway becomes active. It alerts cells to concentrate on growth and not pay attention to cellular 'housekeeping'. Autophagy, the cleaning process for damaged proteins in the body is halted by this signal from mTOR. The cell that has been given plenty of food is too occupied with growing and dividing, it does not see the need to remove these possibly damaging parts within.

When your cells are full, it's like telling them to switch on genes that handle growth - these are called proliferation genes. However, at the same time, many other genes turn off in this state. For instance, those related to fat metabolism, stress resistance, and damage repair among others. You can't have the cake and eat it too!

The Fasted State and Fat as a Biological Battery

The fasted state is not the same as the Starvation Response. In Starvation Response, the body starts to break down muscle tissues (or in advanced stages, even organ tissue) for survival. During intermittent fasting, your body does not remain in a caloric deficit all the time. As there is an alternation between fasting and feeding phases, it does get enough fuel without sending signals of starvation. Your body just starts using your stored body fat as its fuel source, because there's no other option.

Instead of making all fat seem like an evil to stay away from, fat has many important functions in the human body. It helps with hormone control and works as a store for energy. In terms of the second attribute, you can picture fat similar to a kind of biological battery that gets filled up when there are extra calories. It's like having a battery with very high energy density.

Only 1kg of fat has 7,700 calories. The average healthy adult male, having ~10kg of body fat, can store over 70,000 calories as energy. This amount could sustain the adult for an entire month without food (if all other nutritional requirements were met), or it would power the running equivalent to 28 marathons! The human body is amazing.

The Hormones Regulating Hunger and Appetite

It is a variety of hormones that control hunger, appetite, as well as satisfaction after eating. They are called satiety signals, and they come through the endocrine system whose direct approach leads to how you feel about being filled up.

The two principal hormonal components in appetite control are ghrelin which is derived from the gut and another one secreted from adipocytes known as leptin. Leptin turns off your desire for food or it decreases your hunger. It's usually high but not operative in overweight individuals while low but reactive among thinner ones.

Ghrelin can be referred to as a hunger hormone since it drives us to eat. The level of ghrelin can always be decreased by intermittent fasting; this will lead to loss of weight due to reduced consumption of food.

How Insulin Resistance Develops

Inside the pancreas, insulin is made and it assists cells in absorbing blood glucose for managing sugar levels. It acts as a hormone that drags glucose into cells; essentially, our bodies require insulin to utilize or save glucose for energy. Our bodies have a system for controlling the insulin level in our blood to match the amount of glucose present. This means that when we eat, there will be a rise in both blood sugar and insulin levels. After each meal, our body releases insulin which lowers the sugar content in our blood and helps with energy use or storage.

When we don't eat, there is no need for large quantities of insulin. Insulin levels will decrease and this causes stored glucose to be released into the bloodstream, maintaining sufficient fuel supply for our body's needs. Regularly eating meals throughout the day keeps your insulin levels elevated most of the time due to its secretion after each meal. This shows that if someone has high levels of fasting insulin (meaning they haven't eaten anything yet), it's likely because their diet consists mostly of carbohydrates or they overeat frequently during meals.

Insulin insensitivity or insulin resistance, which is the characteristic of pre-diabetes and type 2 diabetes, might be a result of high levels of insulin that happen all the time. When cells don't absorb sugar/glucose from your bloodstream it's known as insulin resistance; this causes high blood sugar because your body can't burn up any more stored sugar in its blood reserve.

Fasting helps to maintain low levels of insulin and improve insulin sensitivity, which is the opposite of having resistance to it. This benefit can also lower the chances of diabetes along with other health advantages. Intervals of fasting may raise human growth hormone (HGH). This hormone helps in growing and repairing body tissues. The body lets out HGH while we sleep or do exercise, but fasting can also boost its creation. Growing older results in our bodies generating less HGH naturally. This decline can lead to loss of muscle mass, which is a serious issue for elderly individuals who are more prone to diseases such as osteoporosis. You can keep your body's HGH levels healthy with intermittent fasting. This will make sure that you maintain good health even as you grow older!

Intermittent fasting aids in muscle development and repair after exercising, lessening the soreness that follows workouts and enhancing recovery from injuries. When we get older, our body's capacity to react properly to difficulties such as exercise or harm decreases. But if we adopt a lifestyle of intermittent fasting, it can assist us in overcoming these limitations by boosting our endurance against physical stressors.

Additionally, intermittent fasting can assist in decreasing the possibility of cardiovascular disease. There are some methods through which this happens. The initial method is by lowering blood pressure, cholesterol levels, and triglycerides; these actions lessen the chances for heart ailments to start forming.

Why You Should Consult a Doctor before Fasting As a Senior

Seniors could experience specific dangers and difficulties while fasting, which might not happen for younger people. Seniors must talk to a medical expert before they start this type of eating routine to make sure about their safety and good health.

1. Health Problems Linked to Age: When you get older, alterations happen in your body that can impact the way it manages food and elements. Seniors might already have health problems like diabetes, heart illness, or gastrointestinal problems which could worsen with fasting. A doctor's consultation is necessary to confirm if any of these conditions are present and how to handle them before beginning a fast.

2. Medication Interactions: A lot of elderly people need to take many medications to handle long-lasting problems. Not eating might change the way these medicines are absorbed and metabolized by their bodies, which can cause bad effects. A doctor can analyze your medication list and give directions on modifying the timing of your fasting period to reduce dangers.

3. Nutritional Requirements: Unlike younger adults, seniors possess different nutritional requirements and fasting may affect your capability to fulfill these needs. A doctor can aid in making a plan for fasting that guarantees enough nutrient consumption and reduces the chances of malnutrition.

4. Hydration: Dehydration is a frequent problem in fasting, particularly for elderly people who might already be drinking less because of age-related alterations. A medical professional can guide you on the ways to maintain hydration during fasting and watch for symptoms of dehydration.

5. Mental Health: Fasting may have an impact on the mind, causing psychological reactions like changes in mood or being easily annoyed. For elderly people who already suffer from mental health conditions, these effects can be quite difficult to handle. A doctor can offer assistance and materials for dealing with such experiences during fasting periods.

To end, fasting can be beneficial to a lot of people. But for seniors, they must consider health and safety first by talking with their doctor before starting any kind of fasting routine.

CHAPTER TWO

TAILORING INTERMITTENT FASTING FOR WOMEN OVER 70

Older women can have good results with intermittent fasting by picking suitable methods of fasting and thinking about their own needs and situations. They also make sure to keep safety in mind for a successful, healthy outcome over time when trying to reach health objectives using this approach.

Different methods exist within intermittent fasting, each having its own way of alternating between periods for eating and not eating. The following are various types of intermittent fasting for women in their seventies:

THE 5:2 DIET

The 5:2 Diet, has become quite popular in health and weight loss methods. Created by British journalist Michael Mosley, this type of intermittent fasting has attracted attention because it seems easy to follow and offers possible good effects on overall health.

The 5:2 Diet is a way of eating that has regular food consumption for five days in a week and then limited calorie intake on two other days.

These two days, usually known as "fasting days," demand people to cut down greatly their calories intake to roughly 500-600 calories per day (for women) or 600-700 calories each day (for men).

A documentary and book from Michael Mosley, is responsible for making this eating pattern popular. Mosley's personal journey, coupled with scientific research and testimonials, helped thrust the 5:2 Diet into the mainstream spotlight, attracting a wide audience seeking effective and sustainable weight loss methods.

The diet does not specify what foods to eat but rather when you should eat, it is more like a lifestyle. This eating method is often seen as easier to maintain compared to a typical diet that focuses on reducing calories.

How to Do the 5:2 Diet

The 5:2 diet is simple to comprehend.

You eat normally, without any calorie restriction for five days a week.

Then, during the remaining two days of the week, you lower your calorie consumption to only one-fourth of what your body usually requires. In general, for women, it's about 500 calories per day, and for men, it's around 600 calories every day.

It does not matter which two days you select, as long as there is at least one day where you do not fast in between them.

A usual method to arrange the week is by fasting on Monday and Thursday, having two or three modest meals, and then eating regularly during the remaining days.

Stressing again, eating "normally" doesn't allow you to consume anything. If you eat lots of unhealthy food, chances are that your weight will not decrease and it could increase.

You need to consume the same quantity of food as if you did not fast.

The 5:2 Diet Benefits and Challenges

For women aged 70 and above, the 5:2 diet has its advantages and difficulties. This method offers a sort of flexibility that is not present in other diets. You don't need to strictly count calories every day but can instead follow your regular eating routine for most of the week, which might be more manageable for many older people. Also, the method of intermittent fasting aids in triggering various cellular repair mechanisms and might exhibit anti-aging advantages. This could be especially useful to you as you aim to uphold your health and energy.

For many elderly people, weight management is a big worry because carrying too much weight can make you more likely to get serious ongoing illnesses like heart disease, diabetes, and arthritis. The 5:2 diet provides an organized method for controlling calories that could result in losing weight if it's consistently followed.

By decreasing calorie intake on two days that aren't back-to-back, you make a calorie shortfall without needing to follow strict diet restrictions each day - something that might be harder for some people to stick with at all times.

Additionally, people who used this style of fasting have shown better metabolic health. It can help lower insulin resistance and manage blood sugar more effectively. These advantages are especially important for you because as one gets older, metabolic function often worsens which raises the chances of problems like type 2 diabetes and metabolic syndrome.

The 5:2 diet could assist in managing blood sugar levels by including times of calorie restriction, thus possibly lessening the possibility of developing metabolic disorders for you.

On the other hand, there could be difficulties related to the 5:2 diet for ladies above 70. The nutritional needs and health worries of older adults might not be similar to those who are younger, so we need to consider this when putting intermittent fasting into practice.

For instance, you might face a greater risk of lacking nutrients like calcium along with vitamins D and B. These play important roles in maintaining strong bones as well as supporting immunity function plus energy breakdown (metabolism).

Moreover, as a person grows older, they might become more vulnerable to the downsides of fasting like feeling dizzy, tired, and having difficulties with thinking. You need to pay attention to what your body is saying and modify the way you fast if needed - this becomes even more crucial in case any negative symptoms appear.

ALTERNATE-DAY FASTING

Alternate-day fasting (ADF) is a form of intermittent fasting (IF) that requires you to fast on some days and not on others during the week. In ADF, there are usually "fast days" when you eat very few calories (commonly about 25% of your regular intake) and "feast days" when you can consume food without any restrictions.

On days of fasting, you have the option to consume low-calorie foods. These can include vegetables, lean proteins, and small amounts of healthy fats. On non-fasting days, there are no specific limitations placed on what can be eaten from your normal diet.

The core idea behind ADF is that when we switch between times of fasting and normal eating, it generates a shortfall in calories and this can result in losing weight gradually.

How to Do Alternate Day Fasting an ADF

For alternate-day fasting (ADF), you make a pattern of switching between not eating and eating times. Normally this includes about 36 hours of not eating, then a 12-hour span where you can consume food, with the cycle repeating once again. An example could be:

On Monday, you eat from 8 AM to 8 PM. Tuesday, you fast. Wednesday, the eating window is from 8 AM to 8 PM. Thursday, fasting begins again. Friday starts eating from 8 AM to 8 PM, then Saturday is another fasting day, and so on. This pattern of alternate fasting every other day makes your body go through more frequent phases without food than what you might have been doing before.

Certainly, handling hunger is a significant difficulty and so is making sure you get enough nutrition overall. It is very important to give top priority to correct nutritional intake to meet your body's needs. This will help you gain physical and mental benefits from the ADF experience. Here's an easy suggestion:

Though it is possible to strictly follow ADF and consume zero calories on fasting days, this is not necessary nor recommended. At SIMPLE, we do not suggest avoiding food for a whole day. The risks of lacking nutrients are more important than any benefits one may perceive from complete abstinence from eating on these designated days. Thus, if you're intrigued by ADF fasting, consider a better alternative:

Turn your fasting days into modified fasts by having about 500 to 600 calories. This makes ADF a bit stricter version of the 5:2 diet but still keeps it safe. In the end, you have power over how strict your fasting routine is. ADF fasting, in particular, can have a big impact on how you feel - whether it makes you feel strong or weak. Studies that concentrate on alternate-day intermittent fasting usually use the modified ADF method and show encouraging outcomes. Therefore, do not think of this adjustment as "cheating" because it does not slow down your progress. It is just a practical way to make ADF possible for people who have real nutritional requirements.

Alternate Day Fasting Schedule and Meal Plan

Now, we will look at how to organize your alternate-day fasting (ADF) meal plan and timing. On the days when you are not fasting, the time to eat and what to eat is more open. You can have your meal whenever you like and choose foods based on your liking.

When you are doing ADF, you might feel hungry too. This can happen particularly in the beginning. To deal with this, we suggest planning your meals using lean proteins, good fats, vegetables, and fruits along with whole grain carbohydrates. These types of food will help to control your hunger feelings as well as keep yourself satisfied for longer periods while giving a continuous energy supply and assisting in managing any cravings or desires that may arise later on.

During fasting days, if you choose a modified fast, stick to the same rules. You will feel hungry in your ADF fast experience, so we suggest organizing your diet around foods that satisfy hunger and keep you full. These should also enhance energy and help manage cravings.

When it comes to beverages during a fast, water is the most important one. You should also consider unsweetened tea and coffee for hydration. As you have a restricted calorie intake (approximately 500 to 600), focus on giving these calories to your food rather than drinks.

On fasting days and other times, think about meal timing that will keep your energy consistent throughout the day to help you make healthier choices. You can try different strategies for when and how often you eat, like eating more food at certain times of the day - either earlier or later -, or having multiple smaller meals instead of a few big ones.

You have the option to distribute small snacks, start your fast day with a meal for a reduced fasting duration, add in a 500-calorie dinner, or keep with the usual breakfast-lunch-dinner routine. It's up to you. Regardless of your approach, tailor it to fit your needs and preferences.

Alternate Day Fasting: Benefits and Challenges

When compared to a low-calorie diet, alternate-day fasting (ADF) causes more weight loss. An investigation was carried out comparing two groups; one group practiced ADF while the other group followed a low-calorie diet. Over 12 weeks, those in the ADF group lost about six to eleven pounds more than the calorie restriction group.

ADF is particularly effective for people aged between 40 and 60. In this regard, research reveals that within this category of people, participants lose approximately five to eleven pounds more compared to any other age set. Gender played no role in determining these outcomes thereby affirming the effectiveness of ADF among both genders in this particular age range.

Moreover, it is easier to adhere strictly to ADF than other forms of fasting and even much simpler as it is compared with low-calorie diets. Studies conducted over 12 weeks indicated higher compliance with ADF mainly because hunger levels were less on fasting days.

People undergoing an ADF treatment plan preserve most skeletal muscles yet lose significant amounts of visceral fat which includes dangerous belly fat.

Additionally, if combined with exercise, there are further benefits derived from being on an ADF program. Research indicates that engaging in both exercise and ADF can result in twice as much fat loss when compared to just practicing ADF alone. Notably, one advantage of using ADF is its reduced tendency for weight regain.

ADF helps control insulin and sugar levels hence beneficial for persons already having Type II Diabetes Mellitus. It has been shown to reverse diabetes-related conditions.

Additionally, this method also increases autophagy, which is a crucial process that eliminates damaged cells and helps with regeneration. The improved overall health of cell may impact diseases related to getting older like cognitive weakening or issues with heart and blood vessels. However, there are a few things that are specific to your age group which you should consider first before starting alternate-day fasting.

One worry is about how this type of eating will affect the amount of nutrients and overall nutrition you get. This concern exists because women who have crossed seventy could already be in danger for not having enough nutrients due to reasons like low appetite, digestive changes or problems with absorbing what they eat into their bodies. If this problem is not properly taken care of, alternate-day fasting could make these issues worse. This might result in less nutritional intake, like proteins, vitamins and minerals.

You could have personal health conditions such as osteoporosis or sarcopenia, and the changes in eating patterns related to intermittent fasting might impact these. Making sure you get enough protein is crucial for keeping up muscle mass and bone thickness; this reduces as a person gets older. Taking in sufficient protein for maintaining muscles and bones can be hard when you limit your calorie intake every second day. This increases chances of becoming frail or experiencing falls.

Additionally, think about how fasting can affect your drug management and overall health. You may have many drugs that you take for constant illnesses, so fasting could alter how they are absorbed, metabolized or work in the body.

You need to have a thorough medical examination prior to trying any type of fasts. This is necessary in order to spot any possible contraindications or risks that might be present.ng them function more efficiently once again.

EAT-STOP-EAT

The eating-stop-eating intermittent fasting system is a type of dietary plan that requires people to alternate between periods of eating and long durations without consuming food. The usual span for the fast is 24 hours, during which you can only drink water, tea, and other beverages with no calories. This method doesn't detail what kind of food one should consume during the feeding windows but rather it emphasizes when meals are taken in.

This method was popularized by a Canadian author, nutritionist, and intermittent fasting expert named Brad Pilon. He came across the concept of intermittent fasting during his study on how short-term fasts affect different body systems in humans.

The inspiration for this idea comes from research that has demonstrated how regular periods without food can result in positive health effects such as improved metabolic health, increased fat loss, and better mechanisms for fixing cells.

Eat-stop-eat was inspired by studies done by researchers like Dr Mark Mattson who explored how intermittent fasting affects cellular health and the length of life. Also, Brad Pilon's method was influenced by his personal experiences and observations as well as other nutrition experts in the fasting field.

One of the main ideas behind Eat-Stop-Eat is that it emphasizes meal timing over rigid dietary rules. Pilon believes that regular fasting can help individuals with hunger, metabolism, and general health. He suggests flexible eating habits.

This permits enjoying preferred foods along with the advantages of intermittent fasting. Pilon views "Eat Stop Eat" as a way of life, not just a diet. It promotes improved food connection and eating patterns. He puts emphasis on listening to hunger signals, and not sticking to strict eating times or calorie counting. Pilon believes that adopting intermittent fasting as a way of life brings about lasting health and wellness benefits.

How the Eat Stop Eat is done

The Eat Stop Eat diet is quite straightforward. You just select two days each week where you don't consume any food for 24 hours continuously. It's not very complex, and this simplicity is pleasant when compared with other diets available.

The creator of this method, Brad Pilon, suggests that you can have some flexibility in the way you follow it. During your eating periods, it is not required to strictly adhere to a particular meal plan. However, consuming items that are truly beneficial for your health such as fish and meat along with good fats would be wise. Veggies and fruits with fewer carbs are also decent options but avoid depending on them excessively.

In terms of when to start your fasting days, it's common for most people to begin after having dinner on Sunday and then not eat anything until dinner time on Monday. Therefore, you essentially skip consuming food for breakfast and lunch.

During your fasting period, you can drink things with few calories such as water or tea. It might assist in making you less hungry and maintaining hydration.

In general, Eat Stop Eat is not very complex. It simply involves taking a pause from eating for a certain time period, an approach that some people claim can assist in reducing weight and improving health. Also, on non-fasting days you need not worry excessively about what you consume as long as it is predominantly nutritious.

Eat Stop Eat Diet Benefits and Drawbacks

This intermittent fasting method, same as any other technique, might have possible advantages towards weight reduction, metabolic wellness, and lifespan enhancement.

The style of fasting where one or two days per week are dedicated to fasts might be simpler for older adults to follow and stay consistent with compared to more regular patterns.

This straightforwardness could enhance adherence and make it more practical for elderly females. Moreover, intermittent fasting can enhance metabolic health by controlling blood sugar levels, decreasing insulin resistance, and encouraging fat loss.

However, this method also results in insufficient consumption of necessary nutrients like protein, vitamins, and minerals. When done for long periods, using this approach makes it hard for older women to get the right amount of protein needed by their bodies to maintain strong muscles and bones.

This might increase the chance of them becoming frail or experiencing falls. There is also worry about how fasting could affect handling medications and general health conditions in elderly females.

Although the Eat-Stop-Eat method has its advantages, it is important to think about your nutrition requirements, health issues, and how you handle medications before starting this fasting routine for older people.

The Warrior Diet was conceived in 2001 by Ori Hofmekler, an Israeli soldier who later became a fitness trainer and nutritionist. The diet involves periods of eating less, followed by intervals of feasting, reflecting what ancient warriors did.

Hofmekler developed the Warrior Diet as a means of improving health, performance, and appearance through controlled eating that appeals to primal survival instincts. However, it should be noted that his claims are not backed up by hard science.

Someone following the Warrior Diet fasts for twenty hours every day and then eats freely for four hours at night. During the whole period one can consume small amounts of dairy products like cheese, hard-boiled eggs, or raw eggs only; fruits without seeds and vegetables only when needed; hydrating fluids such as water, herbal tea, and black coffee should also be drunk during this particular time.

Although indulgence is permissible during the bingeing phase, great importance is given to picking organic unprocessed foods. This plan often commences with a structured 3-week program made up of phases that ease people into the fasting process.

How to Follow the Warrior Diet

To start with the Warrior Diet, you can attempt this organized program of three weeks to improve your body's effectiveness in burning fat. This is a special version of the diet plan:

For the initial week, concentrate on purifying your system by fasting during the day for 20 hours. In this time, feed yourself with vegetable juices, and clear broths, and choose dairy products like yogurt and cottage cheese, hard-boiled eggs along with raw fruits and vegetables.

During the evening window of 4 hours, move to a phase of feasting starting with salad dressed in oil or vinegar then have one big meal or smaller ones that contain legumes (such as lentils), whole grains which do not include wheat; small portions of cheese; steamed vegetables are also included within this category. Beverages allowed throughout the day include coffee, tea, water, and limited milk servings.

In the next week, continue with a 20-hour fast as you did in the previous week. The focus now should be on fat. Start feasting time with a salad dressed in oil-based dressing again, then have meals including lean meats and vegetables plus one serving of nuts but no grains or starchy food.

When you move into the third week, make your fat loss plan more powerful by changing between days that have a lot of carbs and others with high protein. Usually, these high-carb or high-protein days are done for 1-2 days each.

On a day filled with carbohydrates, continue your fasting routine and have a salad along with vegetables, a small animal protein portion, and a main carb source in the evening like corn, potatoes, or pasta plus barley/oats; on low-carbohydrate but rich in proteins, day keep following fasting time frame then choose a salad same as before but add only 8–16 ounces (227–454 grams) of animal protein to it along with non-starchy veggies - finally finish off with some fresh tropical fruit for dessert which is small-sized serving.

When you complete the first cycle, you can decide to start again or make it simpler. The simple choice is a 20-hour fast where you eat low-calorie food. After that, have a big and full meal in the evening with lots of protein. You don't have to worry about counting calories because portion sizes are not rigorously measured.

You can take a daily multivitamin, probiotics, and amino acids to help cover any missing nutrients from what you eat. Add strength and speed exercises with enough water for improved fat loss.

Does It Have Benefits?

The Warrior Diet may appear somewhat intense when compared to more standard intermittent fasting methods like the 16:8 approach (fasting for 16 hours and then eating during the remaining 8 hours). But it's fundamentally a more disciplined interpretation of this idea.

So, we can say that the benefits linked with intermittent fasting are likewise related to the Warrior Diet.

Many investigations suggest that people may lose weight when they fast for 20 hours and later eat during a 4-hour period.

In a specific study, it was discovered that fasts similar to the Warrior Diet resulted in more weight reduction compared to diets having equal total calories but spread out during whole day.

Also, the people who ate one meal each day had a significant reduction in fat mass and an increase in muscle mass.

An examination of six studies done recently discovered that various types of intermittent fasting over a time frame ranging from 3 to 12 months demonstrated greater effectiveness in promoting weight loss compared to no dietary intervention.

However, the review found no significant differences in weight loss between dieters using intermittent fasting and those practicing continuous calorie restriction (normal dieting), showing that limiting calories without fasting was equally effective.

Moreover, even if decreasing calorie intake is commonly associated with the Warrior Diet, individuals who follow this eating pattern could theoretically consume excess calories during their four-hour window and experience weight gain.

Improve Brain Health

The Warrior Diet Is Believed to Be Useful For Enhancing Brain Health. This claim might hold ground, keeping in mind the results from intermittent fasting investigations. For managing the pathways that influence brain function, intermittent fasting can be helpful.

For example, intermittent fasting has been shown to reduce inflammation markers such as Il-6 and TNF-α based on animal experiments.

Furthermore, intermittent fasting is known for its neuroprotective effects against Alzheimer's disease in various animals.

Other animal studies found that intermittent fasting has a protective effect against Alzheimer's disease. Nevertheless, investigation is continuous in this field and additional human studies are necessary to establish the advantages of intermittent fasting for brain wellbeing.

It may decrease inflammation.

Many diseases, like heart disease, diabetes, and some cancers are believed to be triggered by inflammation from oxidative stress.

Research has indicated that this style of fasting could potentially serve as a solution to lower inflammation in your body.

Improve Blood Sugar Control

A few researchers also discovered that warrior intermittent fasting may enhance blood sugar management for people with type 2 diabetes.

Research done on 10 individuals who have type 2 diabetes, showed that aiming for a daily fast of 18–20 hours resulted in notable weight loss and better control over fasting as well as after-meal blood sugar levels.

However, a different study that happened recently displayed how intermittent fasting could improve the risk of hypoglycemia (low blood sugar) even with lesser amounts of medications to reduce blood sugar levels.

Even though reducing high blood sugar levels in a safe manner is good, hypoglycemia might also be risky and result in severe problems.

Hence, if one has diabetes and is considering attempting intermittent fasting, it is important to first consult with a doctor.

Potential Downfalls of the Warrior Diet

Even though the Warrior Diet may have some health advantages, there are also certain disadvantages to this style of eating.

Some People Can Find It Challenging to adhere To: The Warrior Diet has a clear limitation in that it confines the time span for consuming substantial meals to only four hours.

This may be hard to follow, particularly when engaging in typical social situations such as having breakfast or lunch out.

There are some individuals who might feel excellent by eating very few calories over a 20-hour period. However, not everyone could find this style of eating to be suitable for their life circumstances.

It's Inappropriate for Many People: The Warrior Diet is not for all. It's not suggested for kids, women who are pregnant or breastfeeding, persons with certain health conditions such as type 1 diabetes or heart failure, and those doing extreme athletics.

People who have a disorder related to eating and those who are too thin should also avoid it. Also, studies show this fasting could affect the hormones of women more than men which might cause problems like difficulty sleeping, worry feelings, missed monthly cycles, and reproductive wellbeing troubles in some females (Harvard Health Publishing).

It Could Lead to Disordered Eating: The Warrior Diet promotes a pattern of eating that may encourage overeating, potentially causing difficulties for many individuals.

In contrast to Hofmekler's viewpoint that stopping eating is when you feel "pleasantly satisfied," this may not be a good guide for all people to eat healthily.

The Warrior Diet might encourage patterns of binging and purging, particularly among individuals who are prone to disordered eating.

Eating a lot of food in one sitting can cause discomfort and bloating. It may also make you feel guilty or ashamed, which are not good feelings for your mental health or body image.

It Could Lead to Negative Side Effects: The Warrior Diet could bring about serious side effects such as tiredness, lightheadedness, feeling low on energy, nervousness, trouble sleeping, and severe hunger pangs.

Some people claim that the diet does not give adequate nutrients but if you select healthy foods with high nutrient content and meet calorie needs then it's possible to get all necessary nutrients from this lifestyle plan.

The OMAD intermittent fasting schedule has a 23:1 fasting ratio, which means your body gets 23 hours every day to enjoy the advantages of living in a fasted state. If you want to burn fat, enhance mental strength, and make your food time simpler - having only one meal per day might help take you up a notch.

If you choose an OMAD diet, it means that all the calories you eat in one day are consumed during a single meal. Generally, there is a fast of around 23 hours. Fasting for one meal per day lets you enjoy the good effects of fasting and also makes your schedule less complicated (well if preparing meals and eating seems like a hassle to you).

From around 4-7 p.m., it is generally the best time for people to have their first meal after fasting. This period provides fuel at a necessary moment, an opportunity to eat with friends or family, and sufficient time for digestion before sleeping.

How the OMAD Is Done

For One Meal a Day (OMAD), you focus all your daily eating into one meal time, usually lasting for about an hour. In contrast to alternate day fasting (ADF) where there are alternating periods of not eating and then eating again, OMAD is more compressed in its eating style.

Maintain a rotational eating plan where you have your one meal from 8 AM to 9 AM on Monday, then fast all day Tuesday until 8 AM on Wednesday when it's time for breakfast again. Do this same pattern of eating between 8-9 AM on Wednesday and fasting until the next morning at 8 AM on Thursday, having your meal from 8-9 AM on Friday, and fasting until Saturday's breakfast at 8 AM. Keep repeating this cycle for your dietary routine.

When you choose to do OMAD, it means you have made a big commitment because all the calories for one whole day are eaten in just one meal. Because of this condensed eating time, your hunger might feel stronger during the periods when you're not eating. At the start, dealing with increased hunger could be difficult.

The most important thing for fulfilling your body's nutritional needs in one meal a day is to choose foods with lots of nutrients. This means you should emphasize on including lean proteins, good fats, vegetables, fruits, and whole grains in your OMAD. These will provide necessary vitamins, minerals, and macronutrients.

Abiding by OMAD, which means eating just a single meal daily, can be managed. However, it is not always recommended to stick with this method for all individuals. Similar to ADF, it's crucial that you first consider your dietary requirements and pay attention to signals from your body.

If eating every bit of your daily calorie requirement within one meal seems too limiting or difficult, you could change OMAD by adding small snacks or drinks that have very few calories during the fasting time. This way, it helps to keep up energy and not lack any essential nutrients.

In the end, it's all about finding your equilibrium in OMAD that supports your overall health and wellness. Experimenting with various strategies for meal timing and making changes according to how your body reacts can assist you in customizing this way of eating to suit both your unique requirements as well as lifestyle.

BENEFITS OF ONE-MEAL-A-DAY FASTING

What occurs when you have only one meal in a day? The body benefits from the long fasting time because it gently stresses your cells, making them stronger. This process is known as hormesis.

In one Bulletproof Radio podcast episode, Brad Pilon who wrote "Eat Stop Eat" and is a leading authority on fasting science, explained how the stress that comes with fasting can be likened to advantages similar to those you get from weight training. He said: "The body is introduced to small stress that has beneficial effects. If the stress were too large, it would become negative for the human body." A small amount of stress allows the body to learn to adapt."

FIGHTS THE EFFECTS OF AGING

The OMAD diet and similar intermittent fasting methods trigger autophagy, which is your body's self-cleaning mechanism for getting rid of damaged cells, toxins, and waste. Autophagy also happens in the neurons of your brain. This could be a reason why diets with intermittent fasting might help to combat age-related neurological issues like Alzheimer's disease, Parkinson's disease, or even stroke as shown in studies on rodents.

SIMPLIFIES MEAL PREP

For fasting styles, OMAD fasting has its special benefits. If you eat only once every day, you can forget about the worry of finding healthy meals at work or while you're out and about during your day. Eating OMAD means that you need to plan for just one meal per day - this allows people who are on a diet to sleep past breakfast time which makes grocery planning easier too.

WHEN YOU EAT, YOU'LL EAT LESS

OMAD can assist you in controlling your weight more effectively by promoting natural calorie limitation. You will notice that it is not possible to consume all the calories for your day's intake at once, yet you still feel as if eating a big meal.

This advantage acts as a sword with two edges. Caution is needed because if you continue calorie restriction for too long, it might decrease your metabolism. This would turn around certain positive effects of intermittent fasting on metabolism. If you are finding it difficult to consume adequate amounts of food, avoid practicing OMAD every day or try different styles of intermittent fasting.

Downsides of OMAD

Though many studies show positive health effects from fasting and reducing calories, switching to a one-meal-a-day (OMAD) plan could have some disadvantages.

Remember, very low calorie intake like eating only one meal a day could have negative effects. Studies show that drastic calorie reduction could cause higher total and LDL "bad" cholesterol levels, along with increased blood pressure compared to regular eating habits or less intense types of fasting.

The act of having just one meal each day has been connected to increased levels of fasting blood sugar, delayed insulin reaction, and raised amounts of the hormone ghrelin which induces hunger - these conditions can enhance hunger feelings more intensely (Bhutani et al., 2010).

Additionally, when people follow an OMAD diet, it might cause their blood sugar levels to be low or hypoglycemia. This is especially possible for those who already have type 2 diabetes. Other potential issues could be feeling sick (nausea), unsteadiness (dizziness), grumpiness, lowered energy, and trouble passing stool.

It is important to understand that the OMAD diet may not be appropriate for all people. There are certain groups, including those who are pregnant or breastfeeding, children and teenagers as well as individuals with eating disorders who should avoid this way of eating due to possible risks affecting their overall health.

OMAD TIPS AND TRICKS (AND KNOWING WHEN TO STOP)

Fasting for 23 hours is not simple. To take all your nutrition in one meal becomes more difficult. Also, your body may send you messages that it's time to stop. The OMAD diet may require some time for your body to adapt. These suggestions can assist with the transition and alert you about potential concerns.

Decrease Carbohydrates Intake: Reduce the quantity of carbohydrates in your daily intake. Carbohydrates are kept in the body as glycogen, and this keeps you from entering into fat-burning mode when fasting. Switching to a keto diet can assist in this changeover. Try consuming a cup of Bulletproof Coffee during the morning hours. Even if you are eating calories, the fats from grass-fed butter and Brain Octane MCT oil can increase ketone production along with metabolic rate to make fasting easier.

Quality over Quantity: It's okay to eat one meal a day, but only if that one meal is balanced, and varied and provides all the necessary macronutrients (proteins, carbs, fats) and micronutrients (vitamins, minerals). When you fill up quickly with a single food group in your OMAD routine or from being on a keto diet too, it can potentially make it hard to get other important nutrients needed by our bodies. This means that you must be careful about balancing your macros when eating the large meal after fasting for 23 hours on your OMAD schedule so as not to exceed the set carbohydrate limit.

Don't Keep It Too Strict With The Timing: OMAD doesn't have to be exactly 23:1 in terms of fasting and eating. If you prefer to eat your big meal for more than an hour, try doing so! And if after 22 hours your body wants food, especially after a tough exercise session, then eat. The primary focus should be on maintaining your calmness and overall well-being, rather than sticking to a precise timeline.

Body Signals: Although you are taking enough nutrients, it is possible that certain bodies do not react well to very long fasting periods of 23 hours, and this is natural. If your metabolism works faster, you often feel mental stress or do heavy workouts, then make sure not to force yourself into a fasting routine without considering what your body tells you by showing signs such as more stress hormones, troubled sleep, or feeling tired and weak (especially if these are ongoing).

Be Smart About It: Use this method with care. Don't overdo it, especially when you start getting leaner. When you reach your desired results in terms of body composition and weight management through fasting - then the focus shifts more towards maintaining health benefits rather than continually losing pounds on this type of diet plan.

Transition Out Thoughtfully: Exiting an OMAD routine needs thoughtful thinking. After limiting food for a whole day, there might be an inclination to eat much more rapidly, particularly bad foods that can harm you more if disordered eating is part of your past. When breaking the fast, it's important to focus on foods high in nutrients that match well with your health and wellness goals. If you find it hard to manage both nutrition and fasting, it is also fine if you step back and review.

Women Should Be More Cautious: Studies imply that intermittent fasting could influence how women react to insulin and possibly disturb their reproductive hormones.

Observe any adverse alterations in your well-being and consult with a medical professional if needed.

Impact on Mental Health: Not eating for many hours, especially if it's only one meal per day, can also affect your mental well-being. It could be helpful to manage the level of stress you encounter in other ways apart from food restrictions.

You might want to attempt activities such as yoga, meditation, or working out to help manage stress levels. Keep in mind that more difficult fasts may not always lead to better outcomes. Regularly assess how you feel about your fasting routine and make changes as necessary.

If it doesn't seem suitable for you anymore, there is no problem in trying different fasting styles or even stopping altogether. You must also remember that fasting can influence mental health: Be cautious if you have a history of disordered eating since fasting might trigger negative thoughts and behavior towards food.

It is essential to be mindful of your attitude towards food and body image while following a fast schedule; seek help from professionals if needed. The effect on sleep patterns is another aspect: Prolonged periods without eating can disrupt normal sleep patterns and lead to difficulties falling asleep or staying asleep throughout the night.

This Impact May Vary Among People: Every person reacts differently when they fast so what works for some might not work for others.

Manage stress levels through activities like yoga, meditation, or exercise, and remember that tougher fasts don't necessarily yield better results. Regularly check in with yourself to gauge if your fasting schedule feels right, and don't hesitate to explore different fasting styles or opt out of fasting altogether if it doesn't suit you.

Be Bulletproof on the OMAD, but always focus on your body. Confirm that you get all daily nutrients from your one meal. It is acceptable to adjust timing a bit if unable to reach hour 23 or finish eating within one hour. Most importantly, look after yourself. Fasting is a method for aiding your mind and body, but it is not the sole manner to live a healthy existence.

THE 16/8 METHOD

For ladies who are 70 or older, the 16/8 technique might suit them well because it gives a methodical eating plan but not to an extreme point of calorie limitation. This pattern permits enough time to feed which can aid in avoiding the lack of nutrients that is often related to getting older.

The 16:8 approach to intermittent fasting is a type of time-restricted fast. It means that you eat within an eight-hour duration, and then do not consume any food for the other sixteen hours every day.

The thought of supporting the body's circadian rhythm, or internal clock, to help with sleep is another theory.

A typical pattern for those who utilize this method is not eating at night, and skipping food during a portion of the morning and evening. They usually have their daily calorie intake in the middle part of the day.

There's no strict control over the specific foods or quantities one consumes within the 8 hours, so it's somewhat flexible.

How to Do the 16/8 Fasting

The simplest way to practice the 16:8 diet is by selecting a fasting period of 16 hours that incorporates sleep time.

Experts suggest stopping eating by early evening since metabolism tends to slow down after this period, but it may not be possible for all individuals. They also recommend avoiding food for about 2–3 hours before sleep time.

There are three alternatives available for people to choose from when to eat—9 a.m. to 5 p.m., 10 a.m. to 6 p.m., or noon to 8 p.m.

During this period, individuals may consume their meals and snacks at suitable moments. Having food consistently is crucial for preventing high and low intervals in blood sugar levels, as well as managing excessive hunger situations.

Those who choose this method might have to try and discover the most suitable eating period as well as meal hours that match their way of living.

The 16:8 intermittent fasting plan, just like any other fasting method, comes with its advantages and obstacles. Some risks and side effects could be feelings of sickness, headaches, sleepiness or tiredness, crankiness, constipation as well as overeating or developing unhealthy eating patterns during the time frame for consuming food.

Older adults might experience too much weight loss while certain health conditions and medications could make some people need to be careful. Additionally, there's a higher danger of eating disorders, especially in people who have already experienced disordered eating. This underlines the crucial need to seek advice from a doctor before trying this method.

But, for women who are 70 years or older, the 16:8 method of intermittent fasting could give many possible advantages. Similar to various types of intermittent fasting, it is known to enhance metabolic health by controlling blood sugar levels, decreasing inflammation, and encouraging cellular mending procedures like autophagy.

For older adults, sticking to a rigid dietary routine can be difficult. The 16:8 method is comparatively simple to follow and doesn't demand special foods or supplements. This makes it more feasible for elderly women who wish to enhance their well-being without making substantial alterations to their lifestyle.

Recommended Tips for the 16/8 Method

1. Even though the 16:8 intermittent fasting plan doesn't have fixed recommendations for what you should eat, it's useful to give importance to healthy foods and cut down on junk food. A balanced diet involves fruits, vegetables, whole grains like quinoa and brown rice; lean proteins like poultry or fish; good fats from sources such as fatty fish or avocados; liquids such as water plus unsweetened tea/coffee, etc.

These foods have a high content of fiber, protein, and healthy fats that keep you feeling full and satisfied. Also, it is very important to stay hydrated so drinking water or other calorie-less drinks during the time of fasting can prevent you from getting dehydrated.

2. People, could follow the 16:8 intermittent fasting plan by continuously drinking water mixed with lemon, lime, or cucumber to help stay hydrated and lessen hunger feelings.

Limit television time to not see images of food that can arouse appetite, do aerobic exercises that might lower your sense of hunger, and maintain mindful eating habits at meal times plus use meditation when you're not fasting for managing pangs in the stomach or cravings.

CHAPTER THREE

NAVIGATING FASTING FOR A 70-YEAR-OLD WOMAN: DIETARY OPTIONS AND RESOURCES FOR SUCCESS

For a lady who is 70 years old, the main concern is to keep good health and energy. Intermittent fasting has many advantages, but you must manage this dietary technique with caution. We are providing a guide that offers dietary options and resources designed specifically for your requirements. This will make sure that your fasting journey is successful and can be maintained over time.

Choosing the Right Approach

When starting your intermittent fasting experience, it is very important to think well and select the correct method that matches your style of living and health targets. This choice holds a lot of significance because it can greatly affect how successful and lasting your fasting routine will be. Assess your present health and any previous medical issues. Some fasting types, like long fasting or every other day fasting, might not be appropriate for people with particular health conditions or those who take certain medicines.

Think about your regular daily activities and lifestyle. For example, if you have a job that requires lots of physical effort or if you are very active, you may need more energy and nutrition during the daytime. In such situations, a fasting pattern with a wider eating period like the 16/8 method could be fitting for these requirements.

Assess your eating habits and likes. Some fasting ways, like the 5:2 diet, need you to limit calories on particular days. This may not be possible for individuals who like having regular meals. It is crucial to choose a way of fasting that lets you maintain equilibrium between periods of no food and times when eating is possible and enjoyable.

Think about your future goals and what you expect. While intermittent fasting can bring health advantages like losing weight and enhancing metabolic health, it's crucial to be practical in your hopes and know that outcomes might differ among individuals. Pick a fasting technique that you can keep up with over time, not one that is extreme or impossible to maintain.

Prioritizing Nutrient-Rich Foods

Including nutrient-rich foods is very good advice as it can assist you in fulfilling your nutritional requirements throughout fasting periods. This approach is significant for keeping your health and wellness during the time of fasting.

You need to concentrate on eating diverse whole foods that are full of important nutrients. These include items like fresh fruits, vegetables, whole grain products (not refined grains), lean protein choices, and good fats. Whole foods give a variety of vitamins, minerals as well as antioxidants, and other useful substances that help with general health maintenance while also preventing any lack of nutrients.

Combine nutrient-packed snacks with your eating windows for better fulfillment of nutritional requirements. Snacks like nuts, seeds, yogurt, and fresh fruit can offer fast and easy access to vital nutrients and strength.

Keep an eye on your portion sizes and restrain yourself from overindulging when you should be eating. Having big meals can cause digestive issues and may interrupt the fasting procedure. Try to have a balanced meal with different types of foods that are good for nutrients, in the right amounts

Staying Hydrated

By following and sticking with this, your total health and wellness during the time of fasting are greatly affected. You need to drink around 8-10 cups of water a day, but if you do more physical activity or live in hot weather then this amount can increase. It is very important for your body's good work that you keep yourself hydrated because water helps with digestion and metabolism as well as thinking processes.

Think about including other drinks that hydrate, like herbal tea or water with flavors. These can give extra liquid and change your fluid intake. Keep in touch with your body's needs for water, and if you feel thirsty, it means that you need to drink more.

Hunger and Cravings Management

To triumph in your intermittent fasting journey, managing hunger and cravings is crucial to help you keep alive to fasting schedule and achieve your health goals.

When eating during the feeding times, ensure that you consume nutrient-dense foods to make you feel full and satisfied. Such foods are a good source of essential nutrients and energy which can help reduce hunger as well as cravings.

One way is to include high-fiber foods such as fruits, vegetables, whole grains, and legumes in your diet. This helps slow digestion thus making you feel fuller for longer periods at a time. Keep an eye on what you eat; don't go overboard with food consumption during the feeding hours. Overindulgence in meals causes digestive problems which may interrupt fasting patterns.

Drink enough water throughout the day since dehydration could be mistaken for hunger-related pangs. You can also quell your hunger pangs by drinking water or other hydrating liquids.

Finding Support and Resources

To achieve your health objectives through intermittent fasting you must seek support and resources that will provide insightful guidance, motivation, and the accountability needed to stay focused towards your goal on track.

One thing you could do is join an intermittent fasting community or support group online or offline. These groups would give useful information, advice, and encouragement to people who are also trying out intermittent fasting programs like yourself.

Educate yourself on intermittent fasting; books, articles, and credible websites have information regarding this subject matter. Understanding the science behind how it works can motivate you and get committed to following it always. Also, consider working with a medical professional or dietician experienced in intermittent fasting. They can give personalized advice based on individual health goals and requirements regarding this kind of diet plan.

Tracking Your Progress

It means observing your progress, finding areas to improve, and staying motivated.

Maintain a diary or use a tracking app to record your fast timings, meal times, and any changes in your health status. This will enable you to identify patterns and make adjustments to how you fast.

Periodically weigh yourself and check other health markers like body composition, blood pressure, and blood sugar level among others. This can enable you to monitor your progress over time as well as see how intermittent fasting is affecting your health.

Alternatively, you may decide to work with a licensed dietician or healthcare professional who can help you oversee the whole process of fasting by adjusting it based on personal goals and specific medical needs.

Stay Knowledgeable and Inquisitive About the Latest Research

For a successful intermittent fasting journey, one has to be knowledgeable and inquisitive about the latest research which helps in being up-to-date with the new developments taking place within the field.

You should consider subscribing to reputable scientific journals, newsletters, or websites that focus on intermittent fasting and related topics. Such subscriptions would help keep you abreast with not only current trends but also new Research findings being conducted.

Intermittent fasting conferences could also be an option for those interested. In these events, one gets informed on various thematic concerns around the topic through experts' presentations along with interactions between learners absorbed by it.

Try getting involved in scientific studies about intermittent fasting. Partaking in such research provides first-hand information while adding to knowledge expansion for this subject matter's development.

FINDING BALANCE WITH INTERMITTENT FASTING WHEN DEALING WITH IRREGULAR EATING PATTERNS IN SENIORS

As seniors consider intermittent fasting, they must tread cautiously to avoid the pitfalls of irregular eating habits. While intermittent fasting may be good for some, harmony is needed to protect old people's well-being and health.

First of all, seniors should be aware that their irregular eating patterns including when they are on a fast may contribute to malnutrition. With age, nutritional needs change and dietary intake becomes more specific. Seniors therefore should ensure that their intermittent fasting takes into account nutrient-rich foods to meet their unique nutritional requirements and avoid nutritional deficiencies.

Furthermore, in case there is no control over irregular eating behaviors it could lead to unsuccessfulness in weight management, especially among aged individuals. Meal timing and frequency variations can disrupt metabolism and appetite regulation which might lead to unintentional weight loss or gain. Older adults who decide to engage in intermittent fasting should remember the importance of balancing between regular meals containing essential nutrients for normal body weight support under proper body composition conditions.

All these irregular eating patterns cause fatigue levels for elderly persons as these affect their mood and quality of life by affecting daily activities. The instability of blood sugar levels followed by low energy forthwith makes older adults very sensitive here emphasizing stable meal plans accompanied with intermittent fasting. It can also promote a balanced meal pattern as well as mindful eaters within this group.

Lastly, old people need to bear in mind how irregular eating patterns could affect digestive health. Aging changes gastrointestinal functionality hence making older adults prone to digestive discomforts as well as disturbances.

Thus, while doing it is recommended that some seniors take full precautions by deciding the time and content of food so that they can minimize any risk related to digestive issues but rather promote a stronger digestion system among the aged persons.

In conclusion, as seniors explore the potential benefits of intermittent fasting, they should be mindful of the possible risks attributed to irregular eating habits. By approaching intermittent fasting mindfully and intelligently, seniors can benefit from it nutritionally as well as manage weight, maintain energy levels, and ensure that they save their digestive health thus boosting overall well-being in later life.

CHAPTER FOUR

CURIOSITIES OF WOMEN OVER 70 ON INTERMITTENT FASTING

Many women above and over seventy years of age are interested in intermittent fasting as a means towards their health goals. This section will review some regular concerns and questions that ladies in this category are likely to have regarding intermittent fasting, as well as provide answers and direction for them to make informed decisions on whether or not to practice it.

Q: Can I take supplements during my fast?

A: Yes, you can; they don't consist of any calories but beware because certain types of vitamins plus nootropics should always be consumed along with food for maximum absorption.

BCAA which stands for Branched Chain Amino Acids would be one type of supplement that would come into mind especially when working out in a fasted state without taking anything afterwards.

Taking BCAAs will facilitate recuperation and lessen the occasional hunger pains brought on by exercise.

For those who might not know what BCAAs – Branched Chain Amino Acids – are, They are essentially very low-calorie supplements used during fasted workouts to preserve muscle. Regarding whether they break your fast or not, there are no clear conclusions so use them according to your purpose.

Q: Is IF safe for seniors or is it just for bodybuilders?

A: It isn't just meant for bodybuilders even non-exercisers stand to benefit from intermittent fasting as well.

Seniors could see some benefits particularly since it positively affects brain health; also, we know intermittent fasting can help avoid cancer and build a better immune system against all diseases.

I.e. fasting may decrease inflammatory cytokines levels thereby protecting from stroke. On the other hand, other studies have shown that one can reap the benefits of IF as protection against Alzheimer's, Huntington's disease, or age-related cognitive decline.

Q: What is it about fasting that means it can lead to longer lives?

A: To get this answer, the very first thing one must ask is why aging occurs.

Mammalian target of rapamycin (mTOR) controls old age. Lifespan in mice fed a strong mTOR inhibitor increased dramatically. Fasting and reducing insulin also suppress mTOR activity, which is linked to longevity.

The initial research on intermittent fasting and life extension was done using rats in 1945. For instance, some rats were scheduled to fast every third day while others had to fast once in four days or even once every second day. The best results were obtained when female rats were subjected to a one-day pause after two consecutive days.

All of the rats who fasted outperformed their fully fed daily rationing rat cousins. The fasted rats tended to be healthier overall, weighed less, lived longer, and lived happily ever after.

Nevertheless, human beings are not laboratory animals but we seem to experience nearly similar setbacks regarding intermittent fasting effects.

Q: Should women do IF the same way men do? If not, what should they change?

A: Although this question might appear somewhat monotonous right away with most people expecting a 'yes' or 'no', my answer happened to be slightly puzzling because everybody has different bodies, and some women may be okay with not eating anything for 16 hours except for water while there are specifics from the mentioned experiment relating with longevity in rodents that shows women don't have to starve themselves as much if they want to look better than men do. Isn't it all about having one's cake and eating it too?

There are many examples of women who simply skip breakfast and then eat from noon until about 8 pm with incredible benefits. There appears to be evidence suggesting that during intermittent fasting, females react differently than males since they tend to feel hungrier when food is withheld.

You can try it to see how your body react to it. It has to feel good. If you feel like shit while you're fasting then you might be trying to stretch it out too long. There's nothing wrong with doing shorter fasts, you'll still get some results but without the excessive negative stress. Some women might opt to cut out breakfast but have a bite to eat later in the morning.

Q: I understand that when lunchtime comes, I tend to overeat where I usually don't if I skip breakfast. Doesn't this counteract all the advantages of skipping breakfast?

A: If at lunch you notice that you are eating too much then you need to look closely at WHAT exactly it is that you eat to make this circle of excess. Intermittent fasting doesn't mean eating high-sugar refined crap foods. Irrespective of how long you go without them, having these things will only spell doom.

Stick to a diet rich in healthy fats, high-quality protein, fruits, and vegetables. Keep it simple: just eat real food. Therefore when you do so, the crazy desire to consume huge amounts of food in one meal does not occur.

Q: Will intermittent fasting help me lose weight?

A: However, although intermittent fasting can be a useful tool for losing weight, it does not guarantee that such efforts will be successful. The amount of weight one loses depends on several things including their overall diet plan, activity rate, and metabolism levels there are some women who find that they lose weight while on intermittent fasting diets while others may not see significant changes.

Q: Is there a 'right way' to fast?

A: Intermittent fasting works because it focuses more on WHEN we eat rather than what we eat during broad periods of time. Many Americans follow the daily schedule in which they have 12 hours for meals: 8 am – 8 pm for example.

On different days or within a limited feeding window they restrict their calorie intake instead of reversing this pattern.

However, there is no "correct" form of fasting; it varies among individuals based on lifestyle choices and preferences.

I suggest trying out different patterns and seeing if any suit your lifestyle best.

Most of these approaches can lead to significant weight loss when combined with endurance exercise as well as reduce heart disease risk factors; additionally, improved insulin sensitivity and blood pressure have been observed.

Q: On non-fasting days, is it okay if I eat anything?

A: Like any successful diet plan, no foods are off-limits for intermittent fasters. However, we always suggest that you consume more fruits and vegetables and less processed food whether or not you are trying to lose weight.

For a good immune system, eat more plant-based foods that are rich in nutrients, vitamins, and minerals. This action will also decrease your chances of chronic inflammation which is related to other diseases such as diabetes, heart disease, liver problems, and a number of cancers.

While many people go into fasting with the aim of improving their health status; others do so with the expectation of losing weight. We rarely advise that one makes weight loss the main objective of a diet plan since research shows that it usually does not result in long-term weight loss or improved health outcomes.

In fact, mental health is often worsened by this approach. However, if you're fasting to either lose or maintain your weight, even if not, the primary aim is to pay attention to how much food you take.

Some individuals who select stricter forms of intermittent fasting for example eat far more than what they normally would on non-fasting days in anticipation—or as compensation—for eating less on fasting days. Thus consuming an equal amount of calories overall leads to unchanged body weights.

Q: Can intermittent fasting be done forever?

A: The intermittent nature coupled with its variability is what makes this dieting approach better than all the other plans out there in terms of sustainability. Provided you are eating properly balanced meals, sleeping well, exercising regularly, and generally healthy too, then long-term fasting should not be a problem as long as both your physical and mental states remain intact

There's little scientific research or peer-reviewed studies about fasting over long periods but according to studies 5:2 diet often leads to only short-term reductions because people have difficulties maintaining it over time.

The 16:8 method however tends to be more sustainable than the 5:2 method especially because one eats daily. However, even this is not easy since one may fast only during weekdays, and it becomes difficult when considering weekends. The best thing to do is select a design that can be easily adapted to your way of life.

Q: Who should avoid intermittent fasting?

A: Intermittent fasting is adaptable to the individual's lifestyle but it is necessary to understand that certain populations may not be suitable for this.

This means kids who are younger than 18 years old whose metabolisms and hunger cues are still developing. Also, those with a history of restrictive eating patterns or eating disorders should approach fasting cautiously because it can worsen such behaviors.

Moreover, individuals taking medications that require food at specific times must avoid using intermittent fasting. Additionally, pregnant or breastfeeding individuals should stay away from fasting as low blood sugar levels and insufficient calorie intake may cause maternal and fetal health problems.

If someone experiences irritability, shakiness, or anxiety when they go without eating for extended periods, intermittent fasting may not be appropriate for them.

Finally, people suffering from constipation need to do so with caution as the effects of intermittent fasting on digestion vary among individuals.

If any of these situations apply to you and you would like to modify your diet, discuss safe and sustainable options with a trained dietitian or your primary care physician. People with any type of health condition should not try intermittent fasting or any other diet plan without close monitoring by their doctor.

A lot of people give advice over intermittent fasting. However, sometimes it might just harm you instead. It is essential therefore to consult professionals and be cautious when seeking more information:

On the internet, everything you find cannot always be trusted. A person selling a diet plan who keeps telling how nice it is should also make one suspicious since all that could mean is that he/she wants money from you instead.

Numerous websites advertise diets that they claim will easily allow you to shed off extra weight; however, these only serve to empty your wallet rather than help curb those pounds you would love to see gone.

Q: How can I begin intermittent fasting?

A: If you are new to intermittent fasting, start out with shorter periods of fasting and gradually increase the length as your body adjusts. For example, you might start with a twelve-hour fast that goes overnight and gradually build up to a sixteen-hour fast. Also, pick a fasting type that fits into your lifestyle and will help you achieve your health objectives.

Q: Can intermittent fasting help with other health issues

A: Intermittent fasting is believed to be helpful in addressing other health problems such as; insulin sensitivity improvement, inflammation reduction, and cell repair promotion. However, more research is needed to understand the long-term effects of this form of diet on specific health conditions.

Q: How will intermittent fasting affect my muscle mass?

A: As we get older, our muscles naturally decrease in size with time and when combined with an intermittent fast, the process is sped up considerably. To prevent loss of muscle mass do strength training exercises in addition to eating enough proteins.

Q: Will intermittent fasting affect my sleep?

A: For certain women, the way they sleep could be affected when doing intermittent fasting. This is particularly true if the fasting periods are longer or if they eat close to their bedtime. It's very important to pay attention to your body and change your fasting routine as necessary for good sleep.

Q: How do I know if intermittent fasting is working for me?

A: Your progress could be monitored using your weights which includes energy levels and well-being. If it doesn't give out results the way you would like then probably either change the fasting time or else consult a healthcare provider for advice.

Q: How long should I fast for?

A: The duration of your fasts will depend on what you want to achieve and how much you can bear through. People who fast sixteen hours each day versus those who do it for shorter or longer periods are guided by their own bodies on when to stop or continue this routine.

Q: Can intermittent fasting help with digestive issues?

A: Some people have found intermittent fasting helpful in addressing digestion problems like bloating and gas. However, further studies are necessary to determine the effect of this eating plan on digestive health.

Q: What should I do if I experience negative side effects from intermittent fasting?

A: In case of negative side effects during Intermittent Fasting like dizziness, weakness, or nausea, it is important to break the fast and consult your doctor before taking any step forward.

Q: Can intermittent fasting help with mental clarity and focus?

A: Some people have said that Intermittent Fasting improves mental clarity as well as their ability to focus better while at work. But more inquiry is needed to find out exactly what occurs in one's brain during fasts regarding the thinking process.

Q: Can intermittent fasting help with emotional eating?

A: There are some people who have shared that intermittent fasting helps them with emotional eating because it gives a framework and control over the way they eat. Yet, more study is required to truly know how fasting impacts emotional eating

Q: Can I Work Out While Fasting?

Doing exercise when you are fasting is okay. Typically, the body makes energy using sugar and holds it as glycogen in your liver. If you do exercise while fasting, there's a high chance of using up these stores and your body will start burning fat for fuel which results in weight loss.

The idea is to pay attention to your body. When you start feeling dizzy or like you might faint during a workout, it could be saying that you need water, electrolytes, and food. If more suggestions are needed or if there is a desire for an exercise plan tailored specifically for oneself that suits one's requirements best - then make sure to consult with a health care professional.

Q: How hard should I work out when I'm fasting?

A: The top exercises for elderly people to do while fasting are chill ones, such as a long walk in the park or a hike in the woods. It is one thing when you plan on having a big meal after doing a very intense workout during your fast time, but it's different if you can't refill yourself again afterward as I mentioned earlier.

Another perspective is that fasting is stressful, but this stress can be seen as beneficial. It provides a form of eustress (the positive type) which is the kind of stress that improves your capacity to handle more pressure and makes you tougher, yet it remains stress in the final analysis.

Exercise also puts stress on your body. This is especially true for intense training that needs a significant amount of recovery period. The majority of experts, such as Martin Berkhan and Brad Pilon, suggest not exceeding 2-3 weight training sessions within 7-10 days when following an intermittent fasting timetable of 16 hours. Do not forget to think about it before you attempt daily gym sessions while fasting.

Q: What if I'm hungry during fasting?

A: At the start, it's usual to feel hungry while fasting. But as your body becomes more skilled at switching between sugar and fat supplies, you won't experience hunger as frequently.

In truth, the majority of individuals are often surprised by the effectiveness of their body in a fast condition. If you still feel hungry frequently, that is alright. It simply signifies you need to enhance your metabolic flexibility. Keep at it.

IF brings many benefits, but there are certain common mistakes people often make when they try this way of eating. In this section, we will explore some key intermittent fasting mistakes that need to be avoided. This can help you maximize the advantages of IF and improve your overall well-being and contentment.

Eating the Wrong Foods

This is where most people make mistakes. They believe that if they don't eat for 16 hours, they can consume anything during their eating windows. But let me tell you, calories are calories regardless of the window you choose! You do burn calories when fasting, but that gain is lost if you eat without any control during the eating period. For optimal outcomes, it's advisable to stick to a diet low in carbohydrates and rich in nutrition like fruits, veggies, protein sources such as healthy fats from fish or nuts; whole grains, and legumes among other possible items.

If you eat food that is full of nutrients, it will keep you feeling satisfied for a longer time. This can make it easier to manage without food during your fasting period and control overeating in the eating window. Junk food doesn't keep one satisfied, that's why we eat so much of it.

Restricting All Day and Binging at Night

We all have experienced it, working all day without a meal and coming home famished. So what happens? You eat everything in the house no matter how old or bad it tastes.

Think about it, this is exactly what will occur if you eat for the first time at the end of the day. You are certain to consume excess calories in that one sitting – more than if you had eaten another meal during your eating period.

Eating too much at night right before you go to sleep is not a good idea as it disrupts your sleeping pattern by continuing digestion that needs to be finished before bedtime.

To restrict this food desire too late in the day, try arranging an eating period between 10 am and 6 pm. After fasting, eat something light to restart your digestion. Don't overeat!

Not Receiving Adequate Nutrients

It might become harder for you to acquire all the required nutrients that your body needs when you are fasting. Ensure to consume a mix of food items containing high levels of nutrients during the periods where eating is allowed. This will guarantee a sufficient intake of vitamins, minerals, and other crucial elements into your system.

Not Enough Salt

Fasting for some time can reduce insulin, and then the kidneys push out extra water which results in losing weight from water. But with this loss of water, there is a possible loss of electrolytes like Na, K, Mg, and Cl. Don't get an electrolyte imbalance. Electrolytes do many things in the body, so add sufficient salt to your food during eating periods for this.

Remember, fruits and vegetables can also provide you with electrolytes. So, make sure to include enough of them in your diet too.

Not Listening to Your Body

You must pay attention to your body and make changes in your fasting plan accordingly. If you feel extreme hunger or tiredness, this could be an indication for you to modify the times when you fast or consume food.

Not Being Prepared

Intermittent fasting is a big lifestyle change. For instance, you might eat at odd times so it's unlikely that your meals will align with those of the entire family. When they enjoy their tea or coffee break, you are having breakfast. If you have a typical job from 9 to 5, it can be hard to stick with the 16:8 plan. Every other day fasting might work better for you.

The point is, intermittent fasting does not align with usual meal times and you need to consider that. You will have to sort out when you can get your meals ready and also find a time slot for eating them. If no timing is set for preparing meals, it's likely that during the eating window, you might be tempted into eating whatever is available around.

Not Having a Big Enough "Why"

Understanding the Purpose: You need to have a strong reason for doing intermittent fasting. It is a major lifestyle change, so think carefully about it. Be practical - going without food for 16 hours every day can be difficult. You must have a pretty good reason to put yourself through that.

And also, you must change what you eat. To make intermittent fasting effective, you need to stay away from sugars and have a diet that includes fruits, vegetables, beans, nuts, and whole grains along with proteins and healthy fats. It will not function if you consume only junk food within your eating period and starve yourself for the remaining duration.

If you do not have a strong dedication to changing your lifestyle, it could be difficult for you to stick with this type of eating.

Not Checking with a Healthcare Professional

If you have any existing health problems or worries, it is very crucial to consult a healthcare professional before starting an intermittent fasting routine. They can assist in deciding whether this method of eating suits your situation and guide you on how to perform it properly.

Not Listening to Hunger Cues

When you are fasting, it is usual to feel hungry. However, do not disregard the signals of appetite from your body. If you experience extreme hunger or weakness, this could indicate a need for alteration in your fasting routine or consuming more food within the time frame assigned for eating (feeding windows).

Not Enough Food

Not eating enough during intermittent fasting can be detrimental. In case you cut a lot of calories, you might get ragingly hungry and want to eat any junk food available. When very hungry, it is easy to overeat.

For some people, using the windows for your dieting time to enjoy healthy nutrition will save you from all that. You've already stopped eating during your fasting period; there's no need to starve yourself during the eating period as well.

Moreover, doctors recommend that we always take in sufficient amounts of calories for optimal body performance. Failure to consume adequate meals causes poor functioning of our organs which results in extreme fatigue.

To avoid getting too hungry in your fasting window, make sure you eat enough in your feeding window. So this means consuming enough nutrient-rich foods that will keep you satisfied longer. Another thing that can help one is eating complex carbohydrates, healthy fats, and protein.

No Physical Activity

Exercise is an integral part of leading a healthy life and also supports intermittent fasting efforts. Regular physical activities should be done so that one remains committed to their fasting goals.

Lacking Continuity

This is another big fault made by many people who try intermittent fasting for the first time. To maximize the good things about this diet pattern ensure you maintain the same times for fasting and feeding periods each day.

A Person's Fast Being Too General

This is another frequent mistake people make when starting IF protocols or programs like lean gains. The redesigned meal plan should allow as much continuity with past habits as possible if not total continuity. For example, if you are used to sleeping late at night and waking up late in the morning then do not start eating at six o'clock am.

In addition, if someone usually eats every 4-5 hours they would struggle through a 16-hour fast window overnight. Start with extended feeding windows like 10 hours to get used to the new agenda. If you transition too quickly to a long fasting window, it will cause extreme hunger which leads to breaking your fast prematurely.

Of course, you don't have to go by 16:8. Many people report excellent results from following an alternate-day fasting schedule. This is simple; one day you eat and the next day you fast. Alternatively, there is the 5:2 system where you are allowed normal meals five days a week while spending two days fasting weekly.

In conclusion, select a plan that is most likely compatible with your current lifestyle, or else you might set yourself up for failure.

Sleep Deprivation and Stress Management

If you are using intermittent fasting to lose weight, it is significant that you get enough sleep. As per research findings, there exists a close association between lack of sleep and an increase in weight.

Individuals who sleep for fewer hours tend to gain more weight as compared to those who get sufficient sleep daily. The reason for this is that when tired and lacking energy people feel hungry. All of us have experienced that.

Besides, did you know that individuals who enjoy a good night's sleep typically consume less amount of calories than those who do not? Moreover, a good night's sleep has other advantages such as improved concentration and productivity, prevention from severe diseases, and increased immune system among others. A good night's sleep also helps one be better equipped to handle stress.

Vigorous Exercise during Your Feast Period

An effective exercise routine alongside intermittent fasting is essential since it quickens the weight loss process. Nevertheless, an intense workout on an empty stomach is not advisable. So if you will be doing high high-intensity workout don't plan it hours before you can eat. Do not run 20 miles if you're eating time will come after 6 hours only. It is impossible for your body to optimally perform during an intense exercise period with no fuel in the tank.

Eating Anything You Want Fall within Your Window

Many people make this error. They believe they are free to take anything after having starved themselves for some time long hour; however, what should be remembered is that they aimed to lose pounds hence maintaining what they eat.

Facts don't change even if we say them or think about them differently: too many calories make us gain weight but never lose any extra kilo we want to get rid of. So whatever made you fat before intermittent fasting will still make you fat while practicing it.

Achieving these benefits through an intermittent fasting program means getting away from refined sugars and processed foods while embracing plant-based whole foods instead.

Not Taking Enough Water

Drinking water instead of other beverages with calories can lead to weight loss.

Cold water may also help boost metabolism. It has been found that consumption of 1.5 liters of water per day can increase resting metabolism, thus yielding a weight loss of approximately 5 pounds in a year.

Water as well can be taken to fill your stomach thus not feeling hungry anymore. Research indicates that having some water before meals helps one eat less.

Guilt Feelings When You Eat Beyond Your Window

It is common for people to feel guilt whenever they go against their intentions such as eating during a fasting period but it is a waste of time.

Guilt does not change anything.

In case you are very hungry and need to eat something, listen to your body. Sooner or later, if we keep ignoring hunger pangs we can become disconnected from our bodies and develop an unhealthy relationship with food. Remember that intermittent fasting does not mean starving yourself.

Instead of being guilty, recall the initial purpose you had for starting intermittent fasting. This will give you the drive to persevere and do it again tomorrow.

CHAPTER FIVE

THE COMPONENTS OF HEALTHY AGING

Healthy aging means a complete method of keeping good health in all aspects as people get older, this includes the body, mind, and emotions. Here are the components of graceful aging:

Physical Activity

Physical activity is very important when you are becoming older. This means keeping a good weight, staying active, and eating healthy. There are many reasons to make physical activity part of your everyday life. Doing exercise can decrease stress and worry, increase balance to avoid falling, improve sleep quality, and even help with feelings of being depressed. Also, people who do regular exercises usually not only have longer lives but also live better with fewer health problems.

On the other side, not doing physical activity can increase the number of times you visit the doctor, and stay in the hospital, and raise the dangers of continuous illnesses. Convincing yourself or the elderly people in your life to exercise could be difficult as beginning a new activity might feel intimidating. Nevertheless, the benefits are much greater than the first difficulty.

Some ideas that can assist you or your dear ones in making exercise part of everyday life, are as follows:

1. Include different types of activities like aerobics, strength exercises, balance workouts, and flexibility movements. Examples could be walking around, lifting small weights up and down, working in the garden, or doing stretching exercises.

I. Talk about how much activity is suggested and come up with ideas for incorporating it into daily schedules. Professionals advise doing a minimum of 150 minutes of moderate-intensity aerobic exercise every week, plus two times muscle-strengthening activities per week.

II. Select appropriate clothes and gear for exercising, recalling that costly equipment is not always necessary. For example, filled water bottles can be used as weights while walking outside or inside a mall, as well as using a treadmill.

III. Talk about the things you like doing to keep active. Is there an activity where you could involve others? This not only encourages physical movement but also fights against feelings of being alone and cut off from society.

Don't forget, even if you start with little steps towards an active life it can provide big result for your health and happiness in the future.

Healthy Eating

In the process of growing old, healthy eating is crucial for your well-being. Well, it doesn't only help you maintain a certain weight but it also supports your body in terms of stronger muscles and healthier bones which in return allows you to stay well-balanced and self-sufficient. It works so effectively that a proper diet with fresh fruits and vegetables, whole grains, good fats, and lean proteins can also improve your immune system as well as reduce the chances of developing various health complications including heart disease, hypertension, and type 2 diabetes among others.

Sometimes, it's comforting to enjoy those family recipes you've loved for years; however, they are not always the healthiest options. Changing what you eat can be difficult but worth your effort! Besides that, some new favorite foods may turn out tastier than before and better for your health too.

Set aside time each week to cook a healthy meal together with loved ones. Also, prepare extra food for the following days' easy-to-have dinners. Go through the refrigerator – check if you have expired products there. Feel free to consult your doctor or pharmacist regarding any dietary issues including supplements recommendations if necessary.

Active Social Life

It is necessary to take into account you're mental and emotional well-being since it has a massive impact on healthy aging as does eating. It entails keeping connected with others, taking part in activities that bring joy to one's life, and healthily managing stress and emotions. Remaining mentally and emotionally active contributes towards cognitive function and well-being in general while growing old.

Often when people become older, these people may find themselves spending a lot more time alone due to different reasons like deteriorating health conditions, the death of a spouse, or caring for someone else. That being said, such situations can result in social isolation or loneliness which are both detrimental to our health.

It is important to differentiate between social isolation and loneliness. Social isolation refers to having few social contacts and limited interaction with others while loneliness feels awful because one is alone or separated from everyone else. Consequently, both social isolation and loneliness are associated with increased risks for health problems such as depression, heart disease, or loss of thinking ability.

Below are some ways one can be socially active as senior:

- Have regular phone calls scheduled or video chat sessions with relatives.
- Join garden clubs; volunteer or join walking groups among other groups that match your interests.
- Utilize resources like Eldercare Locator which links older individuals' caregivers (to) nearby support resources.

This will help you prevent yourself from becoming lonely as well as combatting social isolation hence promoting better mental and emotional wellbeing for either yourself or seniors in your family.

Preventive Health care

Preventive health care plays an important role here: regular check-ups, screenings, and vaccinations should be carried out so that health issues can be detected early enough and prevented from developing further. Also remember controlling any chronic conditions e.g., diabetes or high blood pressure helps prevent complications thereby maintaining good health.

Here are some steps you can take to prioritize preventive healthcare:

I. You must have routine health exams and screenings to watch over your well-being. Seeing your doctor every year, or more often if necessary because of how you are feeling, can assist in catching any possible health issues at an initial stage.

II. You should not delay in seeking help from your doctor if you are feeling pain or notice new signs.

III. Remember to note down your doctor visits, which involve both regular health check-ups and appointments with any specific specialists. Ensure that you have these meetings planned and noted in your calendar. If you need help, don't be afraid to ask.

IV. Think about requesting a family member for company during the appointments, or to drive you there and write down important details.

V. Keep a clear path of communication with your healthcare professional. Check if your doctors are quick to react to any inquiries or worries you may have.

VI. If you are using any medications, make sure to have a current list of all of them. This includes prescribed medicines, over-the-counter drugs, and supplements. Give this list to all your healthcare providers so they can know about what you take for health management.

VII. You might think about giving a member of your family permission to see your medical records and talk with your doctors. This way, they can help you remember all the appointments and medicines needed to stay healthy.

You will have a better quality of life in your old age by focusing on preventive healthcare and consistently managing your health.

In the end, healthy aging is also about adjusting and dealing with life's changes and difficulties that come as people grow older.

This means getting used to alterations in physical health, relationships, or lifestyle; it also entails finding methods for maintaining strength and optimism when confronted with hardships.

WHY PREPARING MENTALLY BEFORE FASTING IS SO IMPORTANT

Understanding Mind-Body Connection

Mind-body connection is one of the most fundamental principles of human health. It is a complex relationship between what we think, and feel and physical well-being. This becomes crucial when fasting because it can affect our ability to complete the fast successfully and extract its advantages from it.

To be persuaded to do everything in your power to prevent being hungry or bored, you must have a positive mindset towards fasting.

However, our bodies also have significant participation in the process of fasting. During fasts, there is enhanced fat oxidation and improved insulin sensitivity due to various physiological alterations in our bodies. These changes are influenced by our mental state and can be enhanced by adopting a positive mindset.

Fasting also implies developing a constructive mindset.

To achieve a powerful mind-body connection when you are on fast you need to go through the following steps:

1. Be mindful and aware: Practice mindfulness techniques that help you become more aware of your thoughts, emotions, and bodily sensations so you can spot negative thought patterns or emotional triggers that may impede your ability to maximize your enjoyment during this time of abstinence.

In today's fast-paced life, especially during times of fasting; having a strong mind-body connection is essential for holistic wellness. Fasting either as part of spiritual exercise, personal conviction or health quest requires deep wisdom about what goes on inside one's body (and soul). Adopting mindfulness and awareness techniques people can build stronger connections between their minds & bodies thereby making their fasting more meaningful than ever before leading to inner peace.

Begin with Breath Awareness

Breath awareness is a fundamental technique for different mindfulness and meditation practices that help develop present-moment awareness and relaxation. This technique involves concentrating on the breath, observing its inherent rhythms and sensations without attempting to control it. The following are tips for effectively practicing breath awareness.

Start by finding a quiet comfortable place where you can sit or lie down without any disturbances. If you find it easier to concentrate close your eyes but don't feel obliged. Find a relaxed posture, keeping your spine comfortably straight but not rigidly so, hands resting comfortably on your lap or thighs.

To get started in this practice take some deep breaths. Through your nose breathe in slowly and deeply so that you feel your abdomen expand, then exhale slowly through your mouth till you feel contraction of the abdomen. Do this several times allowing each breath to give deeper relaxation.

Now shift your attention towards the normal way of breathing. Feel the air moving into and out of your body as it travels up and down towards the cage formed by the ribs or moves in and out of the stomach region or area near the navel. You may also sense air flowing through your nostrils or breathe touching your upper lip.

While still focusing on your breath you might notice your minds starting to drift away from it sometimes; this is normal and should be expected. Whenever we catch yourselves getting carried away like this, you ought to bring your thoughts back gently without judgments or impatience creeping into you again as you meditate. You may even count you breathing silently, use mentally a word such as "exhale" when you are breathing out or "inhale" (when you breathe in) leading you to remain attentive always.

Commence with a couple of minutes and then progressively increase the time as you get accustomed to it more. Attempt to do breathing in awareness sessions for roughly two minutes at the start. If possible, aim for around ten to fifteen minutes per session; this way, continual practice over a period could guide you towards deeper recognition of what's happening in your present moment along with potential benefits such as stress and anxiety relief or improved overall healthfulness - however, never rush yourself: take every breath as it arrives with an open heart full of love and tenderness towards yourself.

2. Embrace Body Scan Meditations

Incorporate body scan meditations into your daily routine to cultivate an increased appreciation of physical sensations. A traditional body scan meditation may last anywhere from 30-45 minutes. Close your eyes and start at the top of your head, "scanning" down your body mentally.

You can perform a body scan from almost anywhere, even while on the go. However, for those just starting, you might find it easier to begin sitting down or lying down.

Gently close your eyes, or if that doesn't suit you, lower your gaze to avoid distractions.

Take a moment to breathe deeply. Slowly draw breath in through your nose and let it out through your mouth. Repeat this a couple of times, allowing your shoulders to drop and your body to ease into the moment.

Start focusing at the very top of your body. Observe any sensations in your head without judgment, such as pressure, warmth, or throbbing.

Next, shift your awareness to your shoulders and upper back. Feel whatever is there, be it stiffness or a sense of lightness. It is all fine.

Now, turn your attention to your chest and stomach. Observe the sensations there. If you are sitting, feel the support of the chair. If you are lying down, feel the support of the bed or floor.

Keep moving through your body. Take a moment to focus on your arms and hands, as well as your thighs, knees, and lower legs. Tune into the sensations in these areas and become aware of any tension or discomfort that you may be experiencing. Acknowledge any tightness or other feelings without trying to alter them.

Conclude with your feet. Bring your focus down to your feet and toes. Feel how they are. To conclude, slowly return to the present and relax. Take a deep breath, and slowly open your eyes, bringing yourself back to your surroundings.

If there are tense areas during the scan do not resist them – concentrate attention on them and breathe through them. Try to picture tension releasing from these areas of discomfort in our bodies. Jot down any observations made and when ideas or emotions crop up go back to where we left off with that segment of the anatomy. Your job is just to put everything together without trying to change it because this will give you a reflection of how your body feels right now.

3. Practice Mindful Consumption

Being completely present and conscious about our consumption entails taking note of the food, media, or material goods we consume. Release the conscious relationship with all that you access, be it body, mind, or environment. Here is how to practice mindful consumption:

I. Commence with purpose: Think about your aim first before you eat anything at all. Ask yourself why you are choosing to eat it and what you want to achieve by doing so. By setting a clear intention, your actions become more deliberate and congruent with your values.

II. Involve all senses: For example, when eating food make sure that you engage every sense in your body. As you take a bite, observe the colors, textures, smells, and flavors of such foods like paying attention to how each bite tastes physically and emotionally on the other hand. When immersed in this experience one can enjoy more fully what they eat.

III. Have limits: Mindful consumption is also characterized by knowing when enough is enough as well as being moderate in life choices. Take heed of bodily hunger and fullness cues instead of overeating things excessively, because consuming more does not necessarily make us contented.

IV. Gratitude nurtures appreciation: Express thankfulness for the things we consume; this will help us understand better that there is much abundance around us than we thought earlier whether it's a meal, an entertainment video, or even an item we purchase from a shop; thus making us shift attention from what we don't have but ought to have into considering those that we do own thereby creating contentment within ourselves leading to well-being.

V. Examine implications: Just pause for a moment before having something new on board; think about its consequences first! How does this food affect your health? What effects might it have on your relationships? And how does this influence the ecological system? By understanding the wider aspects behind our choices we can make wiser decisions that fit our values and priorities.

VI. Self-compassion: Last but not least, don't forget to show some degree of kindness towards yourself while you learn about mindful consumption. Be gentle with yourself; it is normal to slip occasionally. This kind of experience needs to be approached mindfully and intentionally always making choices that promote nourishment and well-being.

Cultivating a greater appreciation for eating through mindfulness, help us get connected with the satiety cues of our body.

4. Foster Nonjudgmental Awareness

While fostering non-judgment awareness, you should rely on accepting your ideas, emotions, and experiences and let them be rather than holding them with "good" or "bad" tags. Rather than appraising self or one's inner world negatively, the concept of a person being judgmental is to regard it with interest and kindness. How to practice nonjudgmental awareness:

I. Observe without judgment: Merely watch as thoughts arise in your mind without labeling them right or wrong or judging for that matter. You ought to also be aware if there is any tendency you possess towards putting labels or criticizing your experiences and gently bring back your attention towards observing them while accepting and becoming curious about their nature.

II. Practice mindfulness meditation: Mindfulness meditation is very effective when it comes to the cultivation of non-judgmental awareness. Allocate some time each day to sit quietly while following your feelings and thoughts come and go unperturbed by avoiding getting absorbed into either the two or changing anything about both of them.

Thus whenever judgments come up just allow them to pass without being entangled in successions of thoughts.

III. Cultivate self-compassion: Self-acceptance is critical to fostering non-judgmental awareness which involves treating yourself with compassion even more so when you observe negative self-talk arising from within you. This also means reminding oneself that like everybody else, they too have imperfections as well as challenges.

IV. Practice curiosity: Next time try seeing things differently through a sense of curiosity for example how would a beginner explorer do? Instead of concluding things abruptly or making assumptions, investigate the truth behind the experience with keen attention.

V. Let go of expectations: Do not think about how things are supposed to be but start allowing yourself just be in each moment whatever occurs there at that moment without trying to make happenings occur in a particular way.

VI. Be patient with yourself: Attainment of non-judgmental awareness is a long process that requires numerous trials before it becomes part of you so be patient with yourself while on the journey to master this skill. It is important to know that it takes time and sometimes progress might not always be straightforward. Always make sure there's something good you can celebrate about your efforts after every milestone.

Practicing non-judgmental awareness, you develop a greater sense of peace, acceptance, and well-being in your life. This will enable you to embrace the full range of human experience with compassion and curiosity; thus leading to more lucidity, toughness, and freedom from negative emotions.

Achieving a strong mind-body connection during fasting is instrumental in enhancing overall well-being and optimizing the fasting experience. Through consistent practice, individuals can unlock the transformative power of mindfulness, enriching their fasting journey with profound insights and holistic wellness.

5. Positive Affirmations

When striving for successful fasting, one must have a positive attitude at all times. In that respect, the use of positive affirmations as support for optimism and resilience throughout fasting periods cannot be overemphasized enough. These affective tools are capable of boosting confidence levels for some while increasing determination among others thus foregrounding how affirmative statements may be used in achieving one's desired purposes during the fast sessions. Ultimately incorporating positive affirmations into one's daily routine may redefine how they view problems by strengthening their conviction in themselves.

1. Identify Personal Affirmations: To begin with, find personal affirmations that ring truest when aligned with your aspirations as far as your fast goals are concerned. These include reflections on phrases such as "I am resilient enough to fast," "my body knows how to adapt itself to fasts" or "every moment spent fasting increases my resolve."

2. Dwell on the positives: A direct way to include positive affirmations in your daily activities is by repeating them over and over again. Attempt to perform this during calm reflective periods of sayings like; immediately after waking up, just before eating, or even a few minutes before sleeping. Find your internal rhythm by repeating it until you find a comfortable place for yourself either when you wake up or sometimes before going to bed. Repetition is key in embedding these affirmations into your subconscious mind which enforces their powerfulness.

3. Use All Your Senses: The value of an affirmation can be increased if all our senses are involved while saying it aloud. Shut your eyes and imagine yourself as the one described in the affirmations and bring out the emotions accompanying them. As you repeat affirmations out loud or silently, surround yourself with feelings of confidence, strength, and resilience this multisensory approach enhances the effect of these messages on your unconscious mind.

4. Make Affirmations Relevant to Challenges: Personalize your affirmations so that they can relate to some specific obstacle or challenge that comes with fasting. Overcoming cravings, enduring hunger pangs, and staying motivated are some examples of crafting these two sentences to counter any negative thoughts against individuals themselves. For example "I can avoid harmful foods when my body needs nourishing ones" or "To me, fasting is a process that makes me feel uncomfortable."

Positive affirmations are very useful tools for anyone who wants to maintain positivity in life as well as enhance self-confidence during fasting programs. Through adopting positive affirmation practices, people become their heroes who surmount difficulties and build self-esteem thereby continuing their fasts with unflinching determination buoyed by optimism every minute growing stronger than ever before

6. Harnessing the Power Visualization

Visualization is a powerful technique for focusing and motivating oneself when it comes to fasting. It has been found that people can use visualization by picturing themselves completing a fast and accomplishing specific targets to be motivated, focused, and determined. With the help of mental rehearsal or visualization, an individual can program themselves with positive mental images concerning fasting which bring them closer to achieving their dreams. The use of such techniques in fasting can enhance motivation and commitment leading to success in fasting endeavors.

1. Design your fast: Start by designing a clear visual plan of your journey through the fast and the results you expect out of it. As you begin the fast task, close your eyes and imagine yourself confidently starting it. In this case, one should think of various objectives like being healthy, having peace within, or spiritual awakening. Picture yourself during this time energized with new energy levels as one easily proceeds from stage one to another.

2. Employ all senses: To make visualization more effective, try to engage every sense that you have mentally. Fill your thoughts with victory's taste; the flow of life through your body; pride and satisfaction sensations as if success engulfs you on all sides; visualize passing through each day of fasting without any difficulties but feeling vibrant after reaching some goals.

3. Picture upcoming issues alongside their solutions: Consider possible hardships that might arise when observing fasting rules then imagine yourself overcoming them gracefully with resilience at heart. This may include cravings management ability while working under distractions and maintaining constancy towards your dieting blueprint even having some bad moments. Visualize your way over setbacks or hitches for you to keep believing in yourself by showing how much stamina you still have inside just before resuming.

4. Make visualization a habit: Set aside specific periods where you will engage in daily visualizations ideally linked up with either morning or evening rituals. Go into an environment that is quiet enough for concentration purposes without anything to divert your attention. To reinforce these mental images and make the fasting goals appear more attainable, one needs to constantly practice.

Visualization is a powerful technique for fostering motivation, focus, and commitment during fasting endeavors. Through regular practice and reinforcement, visualization becomes a valuable tool for staying motivated and committed to the fasting regimen, ultimately leading to greater success in achieving desired outcomes.

4. Treat yourself with compassion: Remember to treat yourself with kindness as well as self-compassion. Its fine if you come across some problems or setbacks while on your fast because remember you also have your weaknesses that can be forgiven. Give yourself all the support and understanding required just like anyone else would in your situation.

5. Find healthier means of handling challenges: Develop alternative non-food approaches towards managing stress or dealing with emotions. This may involve deep breathing exercises, meditation practices, writing diaries or even engaging in activities like games that bring pleasure and calmness into life.

6. Seek help from others who are going through this: Engage other people who are also fasting including friends, relatives, or any other related individuals who could give their encouragement, and suggestions as well as keep them accountable. Sharing their experience with others who are undergoing similar things makes people feel less lonely thus motivating them not to deviate from the right course of action including sticking to set targets.

7. Think back and learn: reflect on your fasting experience and learn from each fast. Determine what worked out well and what didn't, then use this information to amend your approach in the future.

Incorporating these tactics in your intermittent fasting regimen may deepen the bond between your mind and body, as well as make it possible to have a better fasting experience overall.

STRATEGIES FOR OVERCOMING THE CHALLENGES OF FASTING

Fasting may be challenging to both your body and mind. Therefore, it is important to develop strategies that help you overcome these challenges and have a successful fasting experience. Before you start fasting, think about what possible hurdles you might encounter. Hunger pangs, cravings, social issues, and low energy levels are some of the problems that one might experience while fasting.

After identifying potential problems create an action plan to address them in advance. For instance, if you know that you will be tempted with unhealthy snacks ensure that there are healthy alternatives at hand. Additionally, if low energy levels become an issue during your fasts make sure to include some rest time. Be gentle with yourself through this journey of fasting. Understand that failure or setbacks can happen at times. Instead of aiming for perfection; strive for progress and celebrate small wins along the way.

Developing mental tactics to overcome obstacles is crucial when preparing for fasting.

Setting Specific Intentions and Goals

Fasting can be a potent practice if done with intentionality whether for religious, spiritual, or health purposes. Setting these intentions and goals helps provide focus, motivation, and direction throughout the fasting period. Here are practical steps to establish clear intentions and goals for fasting:

1. Understand Your Why: Before embarking on any fasting journey, it's crucial to delve deep into the reasons behind your decision. Understanding why you are doing this can lay a solid foundation upon which all other decisions about your fast will rest. Take time for introspection and ask yourself probing questions:

I. Why am I fasting? Is it due to the spiritual aspects such as seeking divine communication or religious observations? Does this have any impact on my health like reducing inflammation, repairing cells, and improving metabolic either? Or is it about personal development including things like self-control?

II. What do I hope to achieve through the fast? Explain in clear terms the physical manifestations you would desire after fasting. For instance, do you want to reduce weight, control blood glucose levels, balance hormones, or focus better mentally? By doing this one can be able to set specific objectives and check on them.

III. How does fasting fit into my values and belief system? Take time to reflect on how your lifestyle fits into your broader context of beliefs, values, and principles.

IV. Assess whether it is consistent with your cultural practices, ethical standards, or personal philosophies. This understanding will deepen dedication and heighten a sense of mission.

V. Am I prepared for what lies ahead when it comes to the difficulties and sacrifices that come along with fasting? Bear in mind that you may face physical challenges as well as mental ones while engaging in intermittent fasting. You should assess your ability to handle hunger pangs; social expectations; possible discomforts etc. Approach these obstacles with resilience by way of acknowledging the fact that they are there.

VII. What do I expect from myself during this process? Think of a fast not only as an opportunity for personal growth and change but also for self-discovery. Come up with intentions beyond the body such as improved self-awareness; better spiritual connection or more gratitude. See yourself taking part in a journey towards self-realization and personal power.

Understanding why gives clarity while keeping motivation alive during your fast journey providing direction all along. It grounds you into your purpose making you more committed thus giving significance and meaning to what you are going through. When one goes deep within his/her motivations, he/she will lay down a foundation henceforth experiencing fulfilling purpose-driven fasting.

2. Reflect on Personal Needs: Before starting a fast, you need to assess your personal needs.

This inward-looking exercise involves thinking about different aspects of your physical, mental, and emotional health so that fasting will be compatible with your particular situation:

I. Analyzing Your Health Status: Evaluate your current state of health and existing medical conditions. Talk to healthcare professionals such as general practitioners or dieticians to establish whether it is safe and appropriate for you to engage in fasting. Such considerations may include the kind of medication you are on, metabolic health, blood sugar regulation, and other contraindications to fasting.

II. Considering Lifestyle Factors: Think about your regular activities involving work and family responsibilities among others. Assess how fasting could influence your productivity at work, family dynamics as well as social life hence affecting recreation. Establish if you can afford to be flexible enough with some support system during the transition period after deciding to undertake the fast.

III. Evaluating Nutritional Needs: Consider the thing which is necessary for nutritional purposes depending on what you eat and like. Find out whether what you usually consume gives sufficient nourishment or not while taking into account whether your dietary goals align with intermittent fasting (IF). Plan accordingly considering possible risks that can arise from longer periods without food leading to nutrient deficiencies or imbalances.

IV. Cater to Emotional Well-being: Assess your emotional and mental strength when facing hunger due to negative feelings. This negativity often arises from minor changes to our eating patterns, making it impossible to stabilize mood fluctuations. During these times of profound discouragement, when striving to remain cheerful seems futile, it's crucial to recognize how these experiences can build resilience.

Adopting self-care strategies to combat depression is vital, especially when hunger becomes more persistent than before, challenging our ability to modify our eating habits. Despite the temptation to try new foods, there's a comfort in sticking with the familiar, especially when those meals are made with love by someone dear to us, and have been adapted over time to suit our needs. My recent experiences with fasting have opened my eyes to its powerful impact on my mental health for the first time in years.

V. Assessing Motivation and Readiness: Are you ready to start fasting right away? Look at your past experiences with related diets, such as those with certain eating patterns, and think about which of them have been most successful for you. Determine if you are willing to stick with the plan even when you encounter difficulties.

Knowing what your personal needs consist of will help you understand how intermittent fasting fits into your life and whether it is right for you at this particular moment. All these things make themselves known to us; thus, our consciousness places power into our hands enabling us to make crucial choices that will subject us towards aligning or adjusting our respective strategies whereby we can therefore take care of our wellness throughout subsequent fasts undertaken throughout their lives.

4. Make Your Intentions Clear: The next step is to turn your fasting intention into specific goals that offer a clear sense of direction and benchmarks for you to meet along the way. Setting specific goals helps establish a roadmap and definite results to aim at:

I. Make Them Fit Your Intention: Ensure each objective you set suits the general object of your quickening practices. Every goal must be viewed in terms of how it aligns with all others toward fulfilling an overarching collective intention, such as spiritual growth, health benefits, or self-control.

II. Measure them Up: Define your goals using measurable units to have a measure of progress and success over time. With specific metrics, one can gauge their performance level without biases and also celebrate the gradual steps achieved therein. Turning targets into something more concrete such as change in weight, blood sugar levels, or time they fasted helps put things into perspective.

III. Have Realistic Expectations: Be honest about what is possible within the time frame you have given yourself for fasting. Challenging yet attainable objectives should form the basis of your desires after considering things like where you are in terms of health now, any daily life limitations on eating plus experiences from previous fasts: avoid unrealistically high expectations that can only make you disappointed.

IV. Break Them Into Milestones: Break bigger goals up into smaller milestones which act as stepping stones towards achieving your ultimate goal. Dividing these goals into small manageable tasks makes it less overwhelming and enables one to monitor their incremental improvements over time one task at a time. Every little gain made counts; make sure you recognize it so as not to lose sight.

VI. Have Both Short-Term And Long-Term Goals: Mix short-term with long-term targets to help keep the motivation going strong till the very end when everything gets accomplished during the fasting process later on. A short-term goal will help you reach something immediate, while a long-term goal will keep your eyes on what you are trying to achieve in the future. That's how you can do this.

VII. Ensure They Are Relevant and Time-Bound: See to it that your goals are in line with your main objective for fasting and have deadlines as well. Check if each objective is significant enough vis-a-vis the purpose of its being set by fixing some due dates or milestones that will form a skeleton for personal responsibility.

VIII. Write Them Down: Put down your objectives so that they stick and don't get clouded by other things. Whether as a journal entry, part of an idea board, or even with online tools designed to track these things writing them helps reinforce commitment as well as remind us about the ultimate cause every day.

To give structure, guidance, and impetus to one's pilgrimage through fasting it is necessary to establish precise goals one after the other. It means that when organizing specific goals around an intention; making them measurable; and breaking them into smaller steps that are achievable, we craft our own success stories out of these intentions. Having clear-cut aims keeps you focused and accountable for how far you have gone since starting this phase of fasting.

5. Practice Self-Compassion: Be kind to yourself throughout the fasting process. Realize that there may be setbacks and it's alright if you have to change your goals or methods in some cases. Treat yourself with tenderness and patience.

6. Tracking Your Progress: Monitoring and tracking progress within the period of fasting is essential in being accountable; checking if one is successful; and making informed decisions by rectifying what was not performed well. Here are some tips on tracking your fasting journey;

I. Choose Tracking Methods: Choose tracking techniques that correspond with preferences plus lifestyle choices. Consider traditional methods such as writing down all hours of eating, meals consumed during those moments as well as any other notes. Or Else, utilize digital tools like fasting apps or wearable devices that give real-time data about how long you've been without food including the time you ate last, patterns used while consuming food plus biological responses.

II. Record Objective Data: Write down objective metrics regarding progress about one's fasting objectives such as weight loss/ gain measurements made on oneself, blood sugar levels readings done in the process of dieting, ketone levels (if applicable), and any other relevant physical conditions. These will enable an individual to observe changes over time, discover patterns, and assess whether desired outcomes have been achieved.

III. Document Subjective Experiences: In addition to objective data, write down the subjective experiences, thoughts, emotions, and observations during your fasting period. Notice if you had a sudden change in energy levels, mood swings due to hunger pangs, mental sharpness as well as any changes in one's overall condition. Having done that one can clearly understand how fasting affects his/her whole body.

IV. Set Regular Checkpoints: Establish regular checkpoints or milestones throughout the fast period to review your progress and make necessary adjustments to your plans. These could be daily, weekly, or bi-weekly depending on how long you plan to fast and how often you track. Use these opportunities to reflect on what has been done right so far.

V. Evaluate Goal Attainment: Compare the recorded information with set goals for fasting programs. Determine if you are likely to achieve your desired results and celebrate stages that have been reached appreciating some areas which might need more effort or modification. Use progress tracking devices for accountability purposes and motivation.

VI. Stay Consistent and Honest: You must be consistent while tracking your progress through honest recording of the information that takes place during this duration even when faced with challenges or setbacks. Remain trustworthy about adherence to fasting protocol. Review whether it was maintained or not after fasting periods in line with personal objectives.

VII. Reflect and Learn: Make sure you reflect on your progress and learn from your experiences as you track your fasting journey. Identify patterns, triggers, and factors that affect your success or obstacles in this regard. Use these reflections to refine your approach, troubleshoot challenges, and optimize your fasting strategy for continued progress.

VIII. Adjust as Needed: Be ready to adjust the way you fast depending on what you learn while tracking your progress. Don't hesitate to shift gears and experiment with other approaches if some tactics aren't giving the expected results or when one encounters unforeseen problems. To optimize the fasting experience, flexibility and adaptability are necessary.

This is why it is important to make records of what happens within the body in terms of responses, behaviors, and needs during the entire period of fasting. Defining milestones that matter most within the context of one's goals would go a long way toward achieving this self-improvement. Thus it implies that any attempt at a data-driven approach helps an individual make better decisions about themselves stay accountable for their targets and maximize their benefits from intermittent fasting toward general health improvement

7. Celebrate Achievements:

7. Celebrate Achievements: Celebrating achievements along the fasting journey keeps motivation alive boosts morale reinforces positive behaviors. This is how you can celebrate milestones effectively during fasting:

I. Define Milestones: Determine specific milestones or accomplishments that have meaning for you about your goals while fasting can be used as a self-improvement tool. This could include achieving a certain number of hours or days of not eating food, reaching desirable weight or health markers, overcoming specific challenges, and following a particular plan for a given period.

II. Celebrate Small Victories: Single out tiny successes whenever they happen along the way. Whether it is saying no at a moment when temptation becomes so high; improving energy levels or completing a fasting window successfully among others each achievement deserves recognition. Cultivating gratitude for even minor steps forward is important.

III. Reward Yourself: Use some form of rewards or incentives as a way to mark the celebration of milestones that have been reached or goals accomplished. The rewards should be in line with your values and motivations, for instance, indulging in a best-liked meal, buying something special for yourself, and going to a spa for relaxation purposes among others. Celebrate small wins and multiply the happiness of your achievements.

IV. Share Your Successes: Share what you have achieved with others who encourage you along the way. Friends, family members, online communities, and accountability partners all provide platforms where accomplishments can be shared to make one enjoy their successes even more. Celebrate together and amplify the joy of your accomplishments.

V. Reflect on Progress: Look back on how far you have come since beginning this journey. Apart from tangible results also acknowledge personal growth during fasting such as resilience shown when fasting was tough; Give acknowledgment to that innate courage that dares find expression by working towards set aims

VI. Create Rituals or Traditions: Come up with rituals or traditions signifying key milestones in your fasting journey. Lighting candles, uttering prayers/affirmations, writing gratitude notes daily, or taking part in a significant act meaningful to an individual to show how far they have gone are some examples of how it would look. Mark these ceremonies as part of your celebrations so that they do not remain shallow ceremonials but rather add meaning to them.

VII. Visualize the fulfillment of your goals and success and include this in your process of celebration. Imagine yourself vividly achieving what you wanted and feeling satisfied, accomplished, and successful using visualization techniques. It increases the positive feelings about what you have done well and enforces a desire to keep on working towards your set objectives.

VIII. Show gratitude to those who have supported, guided, or provided resources that contributed to your success in fasting. Recognize the part played by others like mentors, well-wishers, trainers, or medics in ensuring that you remain motivated as well as responsible for yourself. Appreciate more deeply the significance of such gifts while making better connections with other people.

These celebrations produce a sense of pride; achievement and motivation that guides one's next steps in life throughout their journey of intermittent fasting. Hold each milestone as proof of commitment; determination; and progress toward intended outcomes. Such commemorations are stepping stones to higher triumphs so you can make it happen now again anytime when fasting is involved.

CREATING A SUPPORTIVE NETWORK

When it comes to fasting, building a support system is crucial. Getting motivation, accountability or encouragement can be facilitated by having some friends, family members, or online communities.

Before you start fasting, find out who will provide your needed support. These include friends, family members, colleagues, or just people from the internet.

Once you have identified your support network, share your fasting goals and plans with them. Let them know why you are fasting and how they can assist.

If you require assistance, do not hesitate to ask for it. You may need someone to talk to when feeling tempted or someone to help prepare healthy meals for you; turning to someone for assistance can make all the difference.

As you go on with your journey of intermittent fasting, let your supporters know what has been happening so far. Celebrate the victories but do not keep quiet if any challenges come up in the process.

Building a support system is not one-sided. Offer support to others who are also starting their fasts or trying to achieve their fitness goals through fasting. By helping others out with their efforts, your network of supporters will get stronger.

Stay Connected: Lastly, stay connected with your support networks during this whole period of fasting– they should know what's going on with you always and vice versa.- Check-in regularly- Share Fasting experiences – Support each other too!

INTERMITTENT FASTING COMPANION - APPS

Out of all the people you meet or would meet around one per three already knows about intermittent fasting. It's gone global because many people think it helps them keep fit well. But sticking to it may be hard sometimes which is why now there are free apps that help us follow our daily routines without distraction from other things than our eating windows.

Do consider what kind of app you want for your plan of Intermittent fasting when choosing an app? Do I just want something that tells me when I'm supposed to be fasting? Alternatively, do I need it to keep track of my progress in this journey? Or maybe that's the app that will help me plan all of my meals?

To simplify the problem for you, here are twelve dietitian-approved apps on intermittent fasting. They can make any kind of fast less stressful.

1. Window Fasting App

You know very well that you need Intermittent Fasting but still don't know how to go about it; the Windows Intermittent fasting tracker is your solution. It is a super tracker as it can track anything – weight, eating schedule, fasting schedule, water intake, nutrition and mood – literally everything.

Also, windows let you create an eating window, remind one when the eating window opens and closes., sync data with the Apple Health app and Apple Watch, and have a blog on health tips.

The Window app provides visual feedback that helps keep motivation alive so users can monitor their progress easily when they have no idea where to begin.

Plus you will get some enlightening blogs from renowned nutritionists who reveal efficient meal plans that can lead you towards a successful intermittent fasting lifestyle. Even though most of its interesting features are free of charge others require a subscription fee to access them on a premium basis.

2. The Fastin App

Imagine a particular app that can help you with fasting—not only weight loss but teaching yourself too; it is like having such a smart friend who knows all about fasting!

The videos and pictures on this application are so awesome and they explain why fasting is good for you. It also tells you which phase of the process your body is in and how much weight you may lose weekly.

It is really easy, no need to enter your weight every time, just swipe! And it monitors your movements and water intake.

And why do I love this app? At the end of every fast, the app gives me a congratulatory note! This little pat on the back keeps me going.

In the realm of fasting, this app is a game-changer, not just shedding pounds but gaining knowledge too.

Fastin has multiple features to support your intermittent fasting (IF) journey including all-inclusive tracking options such as a sleep tracker, activity tracker, and water intake tracker with reminders to assist you in achieving your goals.

And here's the fun part – this incredible app is completely free to download! Also, there's a premium version with more amazing features if one wants them.

3. Fastic Fasting App

With over 400 tasty recipes filled with wholesome ingredients, Fastic ensures that eating times are amazing.

But Fastic isn't just about recipes. Additionally, it gives fascinating facts about what happens inside our bodies while we fast. And then there are some very useful instruments like a timer for fasting and a step counter as well. Finally don't forget about its cool community where one could connect with other people who also fast!

Yes, indeed there are extra perks in Fastic PLUS although the basic version of Fastic is free. Its cost varies depending on how long one wants to join such a program. When you choose Fastic PLUS, it means having all those recipes; your fasting schedule, and some fun challenges that can make you hold on.

4. Zero Fasting APP

Zero is a helpful tool that will let you know when you're fasting regardless of what fasting plan you are following, or even if you have made yours. This helps to keep everything consistent. You can choose between different pre-set fasting times or create your schedule for up to seven days.

The app is really easy to use with its simple and neat interface, making it a breeze to find your way around. Also, there's a dashboard feature that helps you look at your fasting habits over time.

Zero also connects well-known Health & Fitness professionals who will study your health data effectively and give advice about necessary adjustments in case something goes wrong with the process on your part.

You can download the app for free or upgrade it to Zero Plus for more feature. You can find it on both iOS and Android devices.

5. DoFasting Fasting App –

For everyone, DoFasting is the best intermittent fasting companion. It can be easily synchronized with any devices including wearable to monitor people's nutritional intake.

DoFasting also provides personalized intermittent fasting plans that are designed according to one's needs, in addition to a wealth of educational articles, workout routines, and a vast library of over 5000 recipes.

Given this fact, DoFasting takes into consideration a comprehensive exercise routine for all ages to promote sustainability of lifestyle.

Furthermore, the app helps track calories, water, and step count daily thus taking a holistic approach to health management.

Although the application can be downloaded free of charge, access to advanced features requires a subscription. The compatibility of DoFasting allows it to function on both iOS and Android devices hence accessible to all.

Vora Fasting App

For individual persons, who are engaged in intermittent fasting and require some assistance from others, Vora might be your ideal companion.

It is a simple app where you can monitor your fasting periods, objectives as well as the amount of weight you have lost. Besides, the platform provides useful graphs and reports to tell how one is doing.

This is not much better than having social media. By examining others' wins and sharing them on their live feed, it will make you feel great if somebody gets interested in what you have posted.

Vora has both free versions and a paid one called Vora Pro that allows for more tracking options and access to a community forum. It is compatible with iOS devices only.

Fasten Fasting App

Be prepared for an easy ride with Fasten. This amazing free app for those losing weight while using the intermittent fasting method will help you set time limits for your fasts and track the progress of your workout activities through its smart chatbot that answers questions properly.

For more fun, join the Fastic-Plus community. Meet like-minded people and try cool recipes or challenges together. You will also learn about intermittent fasting generally and see how far along the road you are.

You can find Fasten among other applications in both free and paid versions accessible via Android or iOS smartphones.

In conclusion, intermittent fasting is unique to everyone and there are numerous applications available to help during this journey.

There are several apps that offer various features to support fasting. These features include tracking when someone fasts, creating personalized meal plans, connecting with other people, and providing helpful tips. Some of these apps are completely free, while others require payment. You can choose the app that suits your budget and preferences.

Generally speaking, one should understand that intermittent fasting goes beyond food consumption alone but embraces general well-being in our bodies thus making us feel good in our mind too. These apps make it simple for us to keep in touch with our goals and thereby remain focused on a healthy lifestyle.

<h1 style="text-align:center">CHAPTER SIX</h1>

REFLECTING ON THE SPIRITUAL AND EMOTIONAL BENEFITS OF FASTING

Briefly, fasting has always been a vital aspect of physical health that is highly practiced. However, its spiritual and emotional benefits are equally profound and deserve attention. This section will focus on the role that fasting can play in transforming lives thus, creating a deep connection with oneself, others, and God.

Fasting enables one to reflect upon themselves and other things around them. You become more aware of your thoughts and emotions when you go without food or water for a period of time. This self-awareness helps you know yourself better and understand how you relate with other people. Thanksgiving is also another thing that comes through fasting. When you abstain from eating for a few days, you start to see the plenty around you. Thus, it makes one appreciate life's little pleasures such as family meals or drinking water under the scorching sun.

At times like this, it becomes more possible to be empathetic towards others who may be in need. When hunger and thirst strike at your doorstep, it allows you to understand what less fortunate individuals go through each day as they struggle for basic needs. This change of heart leads people into compassion; a feeling which drives them to make positive impacts within their communities.

A deeper relationship with God often occurs while fasting is put to use by many religious believers. Most religions advocate for the purification of the body and hence incorporate fasting as part of their practices aimed at getting closer to worshipers' gods. By starving yourself physically, there is increased potentiality of concentration deeper during prayers.

Emotional healing can also occur through fasts. Temporarily doing away with food can help us confront our emotions directly, rather than diverting them elsewhere before fully addressing them and achieving inner peace.

The Role Played by Exercise and Yoga in Intermittent Fasting

The combination of exercise and yoga has grown in popularity as people seek to live healthier lives. When practiced alongside intermittent fasting, both of these activities can work together to enhance the positive effects obtained. This section looks at how exercise and yoga can supercharge your intermittent fasting journey, enabling better physical, mental, and emotional self-being.

Exercise and Intermittent Fasting: The Perfect Match

When done concurrently, exercise combined with intermittent fasting can amount to a powerful relationship that maintains a healthy lifestyle. Each has its unique advantages but when they are blended there is much more that could be achieved. In this part, we shall look out for those areas where both exercises and intermittent fasting work hand-in-hand such as weight loss, improved muscle tone, and brain health.

Weight Loss: Exercise is crucial for losing weight while intermittent fasting helps in losing body fats. Physical activity burns calories while also promoting muscle growth whereas IF reduces daily caloric intake. Together these methods create a deficit thereby leading to weight loss. Additionally, intermittent fasting stimulates fat oxidation which further boosts your efforts towards shedding off excess weight.

Muscle Gain: For building and keeping muscle mass exercise is necessary, whereas fasting intermittently can optimize muscle growth. In the course of working out your body destroys muscles as it regenerates them during fasting. This process called intermittent fasting leads to greater muscle gains due to increased muscle protein synthesis.

Cognitive Function: Additionally, both exercise and intermittent fasting have been known to boost cognitive function. For instance, exercise increases the blood flow in your brain which improves memory and cognitive function. Also, intermittent fasting has been found to boost levels of BDNF, a protein that encourages the development of new neurons thus enhancing cognitive functioning. When used together, exercise and intermittent fasting can have synergistic effects on various aspects of cognition such as better memory recall or concentration or overall wellness for the brain.

Yoga: Perfect Partner for Intermittent Fasting

Yoga and intermittent fasting are two activities that complement each other well by providing a holistic approach to health. This section will discuss how yoga principles can be integrated with those of intermittent fasting to amplify one's physical, mental, and spiritual well-being.

Physical Health: Yoga which is an activity that focuses on flexibility, strength, and balance is good for improving posture. If you want a broader range of movements plus minimization of injury chances then this practice should be combined with interrupted eating patterns. Yoga in conjunction with intermittent fasting would solicit more desirable outcomes from both methods; for example, practicing yoga while fasting would increase fat oxidation hence leading to weight loss. Moreover, it could help you reduce anxiety levels or enhance quality sleep – all these being important elements in one's maintenance healthy weight.

Mental Health: It also has mental health benefits like stress reduction among others through its relaxation effect which includes anxiety depression and mood enhancement generally. Again when practiced during a period without food Yoga serves these purposes very well especially increasing BDNF levels during fasts. Furthermore, it could make you more attentive during this time of not eating.

Spiritual Health: Often people view yoga as a spiritual practice, and it can help you deepen your sense of self and connection to the world. Intermittent fasting in combination with yoga can enhance spirituality. Thus engaging in yoga exercises while observing intermittent fasting enables one to get in touch with his or her body and breathe something that helps him or her meditate better. Additionally, cultivating gratitude and compassion is also very helpful at such times.

How Sleep Quality Maximizes Fasting Potential

Sleep has a crucial role to play in the success of one engaging in fasting for various reasons. Firstly, quality sleep is important for overall health and well-being. Sleep deprivation can cause many health problems including obesity, diabetes, cardiovascular diseases, and mental illnesses. When we are fasting we must prioritize getting enough sleep so that our bodies have the energy and resources they need to function optimally.

Also, sleep helps in regulating hunger and appetite levels. A lack of sleep results in higher production of ghrelin, an appetite-stimulating hormone in our bodies while leptin which suppresses hunger decreases leading to increased cravings hence making fast not easy to hold on. Adequate rest can help us curb these hormones and decrease hunger thereby making it simpler for effective fasting.

It is necessary for clear thinking and concentration during fasts. Our cognitive function becomes impaired due to lack of enough sleep thus making healthier choices such as resisting temptations more difficult. This will be achieved by achieving a good amount of rest which in turn sharpens minds thus enabling one to maintain their goals on fasting better.

Practical Tips for Improving Sleep and Enhancing Fasting Benefits

Good quality sleep improves the benefits got from fasting. Here are several practicable tips that will assist you to improve your sleeping habits as well as increase gains from it:

1. Make sure you keep consistent bedtimes: Go to bed at the same time every night even on weekends. Such a habit makes your body's internal clock work perfectly leaving you with good quality sleep.

2. Set up a bedtime routine that induces relaxation: Research has shown that establishing a relaxing bedtime routine can greatly contribute to better rest and overall well-being. These calm activities enable your body to know when it's time to go into rest mode before bed. For instance, one can read a book, immerse in a hot tub, or even participate in other deep breathing exercises and meditation. These activities tend to reduce the level of anxiety, calm the mind, and thus set up conditions that are favorable for sleep.

This routine should be practiced at the same time every evening. Undertaking these tasks at specific times each night will as if make your body feel some kind of rhythm indicating that it's high time you go to bed. Therefore, by devoting more quality relaxation periods before sleeping, your night's rest will become better as well and your mornings refreshed.

3. Make a conducive sleep environment: A good night's sleep is facilitated by an appropriate environment for sleeping comfortably. Some factors involved in creating an ideal sleep environment include:

I. Temperature: It is generally considered best to keep the temperature of your bedroom between 60 to 67 degrees Fahrenheit (15.5 to 19.5 degrees Celsius) for optimal sleep. This temperature range helps you fall asleep faster and stay asleep longer throughout the night. You can adjust the thermostat or use fans to maintain a comfortable temperature throughout the night.

II. Light: Create your bedroom as dark as feasible to tell your body that it is time to sleep. Buy blackout curtains or shades which will help block the light from outside for example those coming from street lamps or rising sun early in the morning. If attaining full darkness is a problem, you can also use a sleeping mask.

III. Noise: Reduce noise disruptions that may interrupt your sleep. Use earplugs to drown unwanted sounds or try using a white noise machine/app to produce steady, soothing background sound that can cloak disturbing sounds.

IV. Comfortable bedding: Acquire a supportive mattress and pillows of the right type depending on your preferred sleeping posture and ensure they provide an adequate degree of comfort. Ensure you change any bedding items that are old or worn out to have enough support and comfort while sleeping during the night.

VI. Cleanliness: To create peace and relaxation within your room, keep it clean and free of clutter. Spread your bed every morning before breakfast and do not turn your bedroom into an office or perform other engrossing activities in it that would hinder unwinding before going to sleep. These factors should be considered when optimizing your sleep environment for you to have restful nights and wake up with renewed energy each day.

4. Limit screen time before bed: Electronic devices such as smartphones, tablets, and computers give off blue light that can mess up our natural circadian rhythm (sleep-wake cycle). Avoid screens at least one hour before hitting the sack or get yourself blue-light-blocking glasses, apps, etc.

5. Say no to caffeine/ alcohol: It is essential for achieving quality sleep as well as maintaining a healthy balance between sleeping hours and waking ones; thus one should avoid consuming alcohol or taking caffeine just prior their bedtime because:

Caffeine functions like a stimulant that prevents you from falling asleep; it inhibits adenosine action – a neurotransmitter responsible for making you sleepy; additionally, it enhances adrenaline release that may make one alert and jittery. To ensure uninterrupted sleep, avoid taking caffeinated drinks like coffee, tea, and some sodas in the afternoon or evening.

While alcohol can help you doze off initially, it interrupts sleep patterns once the sedative effects wear off. It interferes with normal sleep cycles by reducing rapid eye movement (REM) sleep which is important for cognitive functioning and emotional well-being. Furthermore, alcohol may lead to frequent awakenings at night causing one to feel tired and unrefreshed in the morning. To improve your quality of sleep, drinking should not occur for a few hours before going to bed.

Instead of taking caffeine/ alcohol right before going to bed; let us support our body's natural efforts to fall asleep better each night by sipping such soothing brews as herbal tea plus warm milk.

6. Do some regular workouts: Generally, exercising more often is good for the quality of your sleep and how long you sleep. To realize these benefits of sleep, aim for at least 30 minutes of moderate-intensity exercise on most days each week.

However, excessive exercise should be avoided before bedtime since it may lower the chances of falling asleep and increase alertness during nighttime hours. Consequently, schedule your workout times earlier in the day so that your body will have sufficient time to calm down before bedtime. Adding regular physical activity into your daily life will help regulate your sleep/wake cycle hence you will get better rest.

7. Control stress: Stress management enhances both the quality and duration of slumber while promoting overall well-being as well. Sleeplessness can be occasioned by high stress levels meaning that you won't manage to fall asleep or stay asleep throughout the night. Thus, incorporate stress reduction techniques in your evening routine to combat worry and prepare yourself for bedtime.

Try out mindfulness meditation, yoga, or deep breathing exercises that would free up any tension held inside our bodies from a busy day's work. This helps relax minds and make bodies comfortable enough to earn deep sleep. With these relaxation practices that you engage in before retiring to bed, you can have a calm mind ready to sleep peacefully and wake up feeling revitalized every morning.

8. Think about fasting plans: Thinking about fasting plans could also affect your sleeping patterns too. Intermittent fasting can change metabolism rates or hormone balances; thus affecting sleep patterns.

Experimenting with different forms of fasts like intermittent fasting (IF), alternate-day fasting (ADF), whole-day fasting (WDF), and time-restricted eating (TRE), one can find the best approach that suits their body type and lifestyle. This can also help in understanding how the body metabolizes food during resting hours and how hormonal changes can impact sleeping patterns. Nonetheless, you should pay keen attention to how fasting affects your sleep. Fasting at bedtime does not allow some people to sleep while it does not affect others.

Depending on your case, you may need to adjust your fasting pattern accordingly so that it supports healthy sleep patterns. In addition, a good diet during the non-fasting periods helps promote a good night's rest. If you are experiencing any difficulties with sleeping and you have been practicing fasting consult a health care professional to get advice for personal peculiarities.

9. Understand yourself: Understanding yourself is crucial when it comes to implementing different kinds of fasts. Pay close attention to how your body responds to fasting, including any changes in energy levels, mood, or quality of sleep which corresponds with cortisol hormone release. Therefore, if you notice that you feel exhausted all the time, dizzy or there are other signs of health disturbances induced by fasting protocols; it is necessary to make adjustments.

Maybe try shortening or extending the duration of your periods of fasting (how long do they last) or even switching between various types of fasts such as whole-day fasting (WDF), alternate-day fasting (ADF), time-restricted eating (TRE) among others.

Also, if one is skeptical about his/her general responses towards relying on hunger suppressors when he/she has unknown body conditions then medical advice on this matter before trying out such modes would be appreciated.

Remember that not everyone will react similarly considering their constitution and nature so what works well for someone else might not necessarily work for another person unless he/she listens closely and reacts well then one may enjoy overall good health without sacrificing much on other aspects like sleeping habits.

Following these practical recommendations and prioritizing sleep, you can maximize the gains that come with fasting and take care of your overall body health. It's worth noting that different individuals have different sleep requirements; therefore it is important to be in tune with one's body and establish a pattern most suitable for you.

BREAKFAST RECIPES

SUMMER BERRY PARFAIT WITH YOGURT AND GRANOLA

This large parfait can be made for a substantial breakfast or divided in half for a delightful snack. Fresh strawberries are ideal, but frozen or fresh blueberries can also be used to enjoy it.

Nutrition Facts

Calories – 521   Carbs – 87g

Fat – 14g   Protein – 18g

Prep   **Cook**   **Serves**

10 Minutes   *10 Minutes*   1

Ingredients

- Sliced strawberries, ¾ cup
- One-fourth cup blueberries
- One carton (6 ounces) of vanilla yogurt
- One tablespoon of wheat germ
- One quarter of a banana, cut into slices
- One-third cup granola

Direction

1. In a big bowl, arrange 1/4 cup blueberries, 1/4 cup strawberries, 1/3 container yogurt, 1/3 tablespoon wheat germ, 1/3 of the sliced banana, and around 2 tablespoons of granola.

2. Once every ingredient has been utilized, keep layering the parfait and building it up.

OVERNIGHT BUCKWHEAT

This recipe uses rolled and flaked buckwheat, not the cereal kind. Smaller than oatmeal flakes, they share a striking appearance. Stir in berries and agave. Savor and relish!

Prep   **Cook**   **Serves**
5 Minutes   8 hour   1

Ingredients

- 1/4 cup of buckwheat cereal
- Two tspn of chia seeds
- One tablespoon of coconut, split
- One tsp of meal made from flax seeds
- ⅛ teaspoon of cinnamon powder
- ⅛ teaspoon powdered vanilla
- One-third cup of milk
- Two teaspoons of berry mixture
- One tsp of agave

Direction

1. In a jar, combine buckwheat, chia seeds, flax seed meal, 1 1/2 tablespoons coconut, cinnamon, and vanilla powder; stir until thoroughly combined.
2. Add milk and cover.
3. Put in the fridge for eight hours or overnight.
4. Blend the buckwheat blend. Use the microwave for 30 seconds to preheat.
5. Add the agave, mixed berries, and leftover coconut and stir.

Cook's Notes: *Dairy milk can be replaced with water or nut milk. If preferred, fresh fruit can be swapped out* for dried fruit.

CHOCOLATE-BANANA-PEANUT

This smoothie, which is dairy-free is perfect for those with lactose intolerance, is made with chocolate almond milk.

Prep	**Cook**	**Serves**
5 Minutes	8 hour	1

Ingredients

- Six tablespoons of almond milk with a chocolate flavor
- One medium banana
- One cup almond milk infused with chocolate
- Two tsp chocolate-flavored peanut butter powder (like PB2)
- One packet (one gram) of stevia powder

Direction

1. To make chocolate almond milk ice cubes, freeze six tablespoons of chocolate almond milk in ice cube trays the night before. Slice, peel, and freeze the banana.

2. In a blender cup, combine chocolate almond milk, banana, stevia, chocolate peanut butter powder, and chocolate almond milk ice cubes; blend until smooth.

Cook's Notes: *Chocolate Almond Milk Ice Cubes can be substituted with normal ice cubes. Sweetener is not required.*

EXTREME VEGGIE SCRAMBLED EGGS

An excellent way to start the day is with eggs and a variety of vegetables.

Nutrition Facts
Calories – 182 Carbs – 16g
Fat – 2g   Protein – 8g

Prep   **Cook**   **Serves**

10 Minutes   15 Minutes   6

Ingredients

- An extra-virgin olive oil half-cup a quarter-cup of recently cut mushrooms
- ¼ cup onions, cut finely
- ¼ cup of grated green bell peppers
- Six eggs
- A half-cup of milk
- A quarter cup of newly diced tomato
- ¼ cup of shredded cheddar cheese

Direction

1. Heat the olive oil in a skillet or frying pan over medium-high heat. Incorporate the mushrooms, peppers, and onions; sauté the onions until they turn transparent.
2. In a mixing basin, beat together the eggs and milk. Mix in tomatoes and veggies with egg mixture. Eggs are cooked until they solidify. When almost done, stir in cheese.
3. Serve immediately.

CUCUMBER CUPS WITH SMOKED SALMON AND DILL CREAM

Lovely appetizer of smoked salmon with cream cheese, cucumber, and dill, with a squeeze of lemon for flavor.

Nutrition Facts

Calories – 49   Carbs – 4g

Fat – 2g   Protein – 3g

Prep   **Cook**   **Serves**

30 Minutes   15 Minutes   12

Ingredients

- 24 cucmber slices, approximately 3/4-inch thick each
- Four ounces of softened cream cheese
- Two tablespoons of freshly chopped dill
- One tsp lemon zest
- ½ tsp freshly squeezed lemon juice
- ¼ teaspoon of black pepper, ground
- Four ounces of smoked salmon, sliced into two-inch pieces

Direction

1. Using a melon baller, make a 1/2-inch-deep depression on one side of each cucumber slice to form a cup. After scooping the sides, place the cucumbers on paper towels to drain for fifteen minutes.
2. In a bowl, thoroughly mix cream cheese, chopped dill, lemon zest, lemon juice, and pepper.
3. Divide the cheese mixture into each cucumber cup using about 1/2 teaspoon. Place a strip of salmon and a dill sprig on top of each cup.

Recipe Tips: *If preferred, you can use reduced-fat cream cheese and replace the smoked salmon with smoked trout. You can put together cucumber cups up to 24 hours before serving. Simply store them in a*

BANANA PANCAKES

Delicious, homemade banana pancakes that will please a large crowd in a matter of minutes. An excellent take on regular pancakes.

Nutrition Facts

Calories – 193   Carbs – 7g

Fat – 29g   Protein – 5g

Prep   **Cook**   **Serves**

5 Minutes   10 Minutes   6

Ingredients

- 1 cup flour (all-purpose)
- One spoonful of powdered sugar two tsp powdered baking
- One-half teaspoon of salt
- One beaten egg
- One cup of milk
- Two tsp of vegetable oil
- Two ripe, mashed bananas

Direction

1. Compile every component.
2. In a bowl, mix together flour, white sugar, baking powder, and salt. Beat the egg, milk, vegetable oil, and bananas together in another bowl.
3. Mix the flour mixture into the banana mixture; a slightly lumpy batter will result.
4. Heat a frying pan or griddle that has been lightly greased over medium-high heat.
5. Using about 1/4 cup of batter for each pancake, pour or scoop the mixture onto the griddle.
6. Cook for 3 to 5 minutes on each side, or until pancakes are golden brown.
7. Enjoy and serve hot.

CURRIED CASHEW, PEAR, AND GRAPE SALAD

This salad with cashews and pears is known as The Good Salad. People always ask me for the recipe when I cook this salad for them. My family makes similar requests every time.

Prep   ***Cook***   ***Serves***

30 Minutes   *15 Minutes*   6

Ingredients

- ¾ cup cashew halves
- Four bacon pieces, roughly diced
- One tablespoon of melted butter
- One tsp finely chopped, fresh rosemary
- One tsp curry powder
- One-third cup brown sugar
- A smidgeon of kosher salt
- One-half teaspoon of cayenne

Getting dressed:

- Three tsp white wine vinegar ,three, tsp Dijon mustard, two tsp honey and half a cup of olive oil
- To taste, add salt and black pepper, a salad
- One 10-oz packet of blended salad greens, ½ medium-sized Bosc pear, cut thinly and half a cup of seedless red grapes

Direction

3. In a big bowl, arrange 1/4 cup blueberries, 1/4 cup strawberries, 1/3 container yogurt, 1/3 tablespoon wheat germ, 1/3 of the sliced banana, and around 2 tablespoons of granola.

4. Once every ingredient has been utilized, keep layering the parfait and building it up.

MEATLESS SWEET POTATO BURRITO BOWL

The earthy sweetness of roasted sweet potatoes paired with flavorful black beans and topped with sautéed poblano peppers, red bell peppers, and onions elevate this plant-based burrito bowl to a whole new level of deliciousness. Add some fresh cilantro and a lime on top.

Prep   **Cook**   **Serves**

15 Minutes   20 Minutes   4

Ingredients

- 1 chopped and peeled sweet potato
- One yellow onion
- Two teaspoons, divided, of grapeseed oil
- One fifteen-ounce can of rinsed and drained black beans
- One box (1 ounce) of split taco seasoning
- ½ cup chopped tomatoes cooked over fire
- ½ sliced poblano pepper
- One sliced red bell pepper
- Four cups of freshly cooked, heated rice

Direction

1. Set the oven's temperature to 400°F, or 200°C. Spread the sweet potatoes equally on a baking sheet.
2. Bake sweet potatoes for 15 to 20 minutes, or until they are soft. Place aside and allow to cool.
3. Meanwhile, chop the other half of the yellow onion and slice half of it, setting it aside.
4. In a pot, warm up one tablespoon of grape seed oil over medium-high heat. For two to three minutes, add the chopped onions and simmer. Stir in 1/2 of the taco spice packet and the beans. Simmer the beans for fifteen minutes after adding the fire-roasted tomatoes and lowering the heat.
5. Meanwhile, place the leftover grape seed oil in a skillet and heat it to medium. Add the red Bell pepper, poblano, and cut yellow onions. After thoroughly mixing, add the remaining taco
6. Spice packet and swirl to blend the flavors. Simmer the mixture for 5-7 minutes.
7. Place the cooked rice in a bowl and top with the black bean mixture, sautéed onions,
8. Poblano, and red bell peppers, and roasted sweet potatoes.

MEATLESS SWEET POTATO

BURRITO BOWL

Avocado toast, can be a whole meal when you top it with an egg. Occasionally, you can flavor the avocado with balsamic vinegar rather than lemon juice. The egg can be fried or poached.

Nutrition Facts

Calories – 321   Carbs – 23g

Fat – 21g   Protein – 12g

Prep   **Cook**   **Serves**

5 Minutes   5 Minutes   2

Ingredients

- One tsp of butter
- Two eggs
- Two pieces of multigrain bread
- One ripe avocado, peeled and pitted
- One tsp lemon juice, or more to taste
- One cayenne pepper pinch
- To taste sea salt
- To taste, grind black pepper

Direction

1. Melt the butter in a pan over medium-low heat. Separate the eggs into the skillet and cook for two to three minutes, or until the bottom layer of the eggs is white and the eggs are hard enough to turn over.

2. Eggs should be cooked for a further two to five minutes after being flipped, being careful not to break the yolk.

3. Toast the bread pieces for three to five minutes, or until they are done.

4. In a bowl, mash the avocado and add the lemon juice, sea salt, and cayenne.

5. Toast is topped with the avocado mixture. Add a fried egg on top and season with pepper and sea salt.

CINNAMON-PEACH COTTAGE CHEESE PANCAKES

A pancake made with cottage cheese and fruit for taste.

Prep   **Cook**   **Serves**

10 Minutes   30 Minutes   4

Ingredients

- 4 eggs
- One cup cottage cheese
- Half a cup of milk
- One tsp vanilla essence
- Two tablespoons of melted butter
- One shredded peach
- One cup of flour for all purposes
- Two tsp of white sugar
- One pinch of salt
- One-half teaspoon of baking soda
- One tsp finely ground cinnamon

Direction

1. In a large bowl, combine eggs, cottage cheese, milk, butter, vanilla, and peach.
2. In a separate bowl, mix together flour, sugar, salt, baking soda, and cinnamon. Just combine the flour mixture with the cottage cheese mixture by stirring.
3. Put a griddle over medium-high heat with a light oil coating.
4. Spoon the batter onto the griddle in generous portions, and heat until bubbles appear and the edges become crispy. Cook until the opposite side is browned after flipping. Proceed with the leftover batter.

LUNCH RECIPES

HIGH-PROTEIN VEGAN STIR-FRY

This is a tasty, high-protein, plant-based recipe that can be modified to fit your pantry using ingredients like tofu, sweet potatoes, and quinoa. You are welcome to add a few handfuls of your preferred vegetables or tempeh or another plant-based protein in place of the tofu.

Prep   **Cook**   **Serves**

20 Minutes   35Minutes   2

Ingredients

- ½ package (12 ounces) extra-firm tofu
- Half a cup low-sodium soy sauce
- One-third cup agave nectar
- One spoonful of mustard dijon
- One-half teaspoon of ground ginger
- 1/4 tsp sesame oil
- One cayenne pepper pinch, or to taste
- One cup of water
- ½ cup of raw quinoa
- Peel and cube one sweet potato, or more to taste

Direction

1. Place the tofu on a cutting board and cover with two layers of folded dish towels. Top with another two folded dishtowels and a thick book. For at least five to ten minutes, press the tofu. Cube into small pieces.

2. A big nonstick pan should be heated to medium heat. Add the tofu and dry-fry for about five minutes, or until browned on one side.

3. Cook for a further five minutes after flipping, or until the opposite side is golden.

Ingredients

One sliced onion

Two tsp of peanut oil

Cook's Notes:

You can substitute 1/2 teaspoon dry mustard for the Dijon, liquid aminos for the soy sauce, cayenne for chili powder, agave for maple syrup or honey (in non-vegan recipes), and soy sauce for chili powder. A red onion can also be used in place of the white onion, if you'd like.

If you like, add a handful of almonds, cashews, peanuts, walnuts, or a blend of nuts at the end of cooking.

Direction

4. As the tofu is cooking, combine the soy sauce, ginger, sesame oil, agave nectar, Dijon mustard, and cayenne pepper in a bowl. Add the fried tofu and toss well to cover it in marinade. Refrigerate the bowl for at least thirty minutes with a cover on.

5. Bring the water and quinoa together in a small saucepan to a boil. After quinoa is frothy and the water has been absorbed, reduce heat to medium and simmer for 13 to 15 minutes.

6. While the quinoa cooks, keep an eye on it and add more water as needed.

7. Sweet potatoes should be placed in a small saucepan with one or two inches of water on top while the quinoa is cooking. After coming to a boil, cook for three minutes. Empty.

8. In a large frying pan over medium-high heat, combine cooked quinoa, tofu and marinade, cooked sweet potatoes, onion, and peanut oil. Cook for 3 to 4 minutes, stirring continuously, or until onion is tender.

VEGETARIAN REFRIED BEANS

Delicious traditional vegetarian and vegan refried beans with very little fat!

Prep   **Cook**   **Serves**

15 Minutes   4 hour   12

Ingredients

- 1 pound of rinsed and dry pinto beans
- Two tsp finely chopped garlic, split
- One medium tomato, chopped
- Two tsp finely ground cumin
- One tablespoon of powdered chilies
- Two tsp olive oil
- Salt according to taste

Direction

1. Put the beans in a big pot and add one inch of water to cover them. Elevate the temperature to a boiling point. After the beans reach a boiling point, drain and put them back in the same pot.

2. Add 2 inches of water to the beans and toss in 1 tablespoon each of tomato, garlic, cumin, and chili powder. Bring to a boil over high heat, then lower the heat to a simmer and cook, stirring occasionally, until the beans are very tender, about 3 hours and 45 minutes.

3. After the beans are done, mash them with the oil, salt, and remaining garlic; add water as necessary to get the right consistency. After 30 minutes of low heat, stir occasionally.

BUDDHA BOWL

Delicious and healthful dinner in less than an hour

<table>
<tr><td>**Prep**</td><td>**Cook**</td><td>**Serves**</td></tr>
<tr><td>10 Minutes</td><td>48 hour</td><td>4</td></tr>
</table>

Ingredients

- Three cups of chicken stock
- One and a half cups quinoa
- One big sweet potato, chopped
- One big red onion, chopped
- Split ¼ cup of olive oil.
- Taste-tested kosher salt
- Freshly ground black pepper according to taste

Direction

1. In a saucepan, bring the quinoa and chicken broth to a boil. After 15 to 20 minutes, or until the quinoa is soft and the stock has been absorbed, reduce heat to medium-low, cover, and simmer.
2. Set oven temperature to 425 F (220 C).
3. Arrange the red onion and sweet potato on a baking pan. Pour one tablespoon of olive oil over the mixture, add salt and pepper, and toss to coat.
4. Bake for 20 to 25 minutes, or until sweet potatoes are soft, in a preheated oven.

Ingredients

- Three minced garlic cloves, divided
- One tablespoon of freshly chopped ginger root
- One-pound portions of skinless, boneless chicken breasts
- 1/4 cup lime juice
- Two teaspoons of creamy peanut butter
- One spoonful of soy sauce
- One tablespoon of honey
- One tablespoon of sesame oil
- two cups of baby spinach
- One avocado, thinly cut, pitted, and peeled
- One tablespoon of freshly cut cilantro
- One teaspoon of sesame seeds, roasted

Direction

5. One tablespoon of olive oil should be heated in a skillet over medium heat. Cook and stir 2 cloves of garlic and ginger for about 1 minute, or until fragrant.

6. When the chicken is no longer pink in the middle and its juices run clear, add it and cook it for about 6 minutes on each side. An instant-read thermometer should read at least 165 degrees Fahrenheit (74 degrees Celsius) when positioned in the center. Chop the chicken until it is in 1-inch pieces.

7. In a bowl, whisk together 1 clove garlic, lime juice, peanut butter, soy sauce, and honey.

8. Blend the mixture with 1 tablespoon of olive oil and sesame oil until a creamy dressing is achieved.

9. Spoon quinoa into each bowl; add avocado, spinach, sweet potato mixture, and chicken on top. Drizzle dressing over each bowl and garnish with sesame seeds and cilantro.

YUMMY VEGGIE OMELET

Serve this delightful vegetarian omelet over bread. Choose your favorite cheese; Gouda and Swiss are both excellent options.

Prep   **Cook**   **Serves**

10 Minutes   10 minutes   2

Ingredients

- Two tablespoons of butter, separated
- One little onion, finely sliced
- One sliced green bell pepper
- 1/4 tsp salt, separated
- Four big eggs
- two tsp milk
- One-third of a teaspoon freshly ground pepper
- Two ounces of Swiss cheese, shredded

Direction

1. In a medium pan set over medium heat, melt 1 tablespoon of butter. In butter, cook and toss onion and bell pepper for 4 to 5 minutes, or until they are just soft. Move the veggies into a bowl, sprinkle with 1/4 tsp salt, and reserve.

2. In a separate bowl, beat together eggs, milk, pepper, and the remaining 1/2 teaspoon salt.

3. In the skillet over medium heat, melt the remaining tablespoon of butter and swirl to coat the bottom of the pan. Pour in egg mixture and heat, stirring occasionally, until bottoms of eggs start to set, about 1 minute, after butter has melted.

Ingredients

Direction

4. Using a spatula, gently lift the omelet's edges so that any egg that isn't cooked can spill onto the skillet. Cook for an additional one to two minutes, or until the middle of the omelet begins to look dry.
5. After sprinkling the omelet with cheese, spread the veggie mixture over half of it.
6. Gently fold omelet over vegetables with spatula. Simmer for about a minute, or until cheese melts to the desired consistency. Transfer the omelet to a dish. Slice in half and present.

CHICKEN SALAD WRAPS

Delicious sandwich for a picnic or lunch, with a salsa twist. Add some finely chopped jalapeño Chile peppers for an even spicier variation! That concludes the matter!

Prep   **Cook**   **Serves**

10 Minutes   10 Minutes   6

Ingredients

- 2 (10-oz) cans of chunky, drained, and flaked chicken
- Half a cup finely chopped onion
- Half a cup of mayonnaise
- four tsp of new salsa
- To taste, add salt and pepper.
- Six flour tortillas (10 inches)
- Twelve lettuce leaves

Direction

1. Combine the chicken, onion, salsa, mayonnaise, salt, and pepper in a small bowl.
2. Combine thoroughly.
3. Lay down two lettuce leaves on each tortilla, then evenly distribute the chicken salad mixture over them.
4. Roll each tortilla up, or "wrap."

CHOCOLATE CHIP CINNAMON COOKIES

Sweet chocolate chip cookies with a hint of spice.

Prep　　**Cook**　　**Serves**
30 Minutes　*10 Minutes*　　12

Ingredients

- one cup softened butter
- ½ cup of ultrafine sugar
- Half a cup of light brown sugar
- One tsp vanilla essence
- two eggs
- a half-cup of all-purpose flour
- One tsp baking soda
- Half a teaspoon of salt
- One tsp of cinnamon

Direction

1. Assign 350 F (175 C) as the oven temperature.
2. Creamy and smooth butter, brown sugar, confectioners' sugar, and vanilla should be combined in a medium-sized bowl.
3. Beat in the eggs. Combine the flour, baking soda, salt, cinnamon, and pudding mix in a big bowl.
4. Until fully combined, gradually stir the dry ingredients into the creamy mixture.
5. Add chocolate chips and nuts (if using) and stir.
6. Drop onto ungreased baking sheets by teaspoonful spaced two inches apart.

Ingredients

Direction

7. Bake for 8 to 10 minutes, or until golden brown, in a preheated oven.
8. Take out of the oven and let the cookies cool down a little bit on the baking sheets before transferring them to wire racks to finish cooling.

FARMER'S MARKET VEGETARIAN QUESADILLAS

These quesadillas, which make the most of straightforward, fresh ingredients from your neighborhood Farmer's Market, are excellent as light bites or a quick and nutritious dinner.

Nutrition Facts

Calories – 161   Carbs – 87g

Fat – 25g   Protein – 9g

Prep   **Cook**   **Serves**

15 Minutes   15 Minutes   6

Ingredients

- ½ cup finely sliced red pepper
- ½ cup finely sliced zucchini
- Chopped yellow squash, ½ cup
- ½ cup finely cut red onion
- Half a cup of finely chopped mushrooms
- One tablespoon of olive oil
- cooking oil

Direction

1. Combine red pepper, zucchini, yellow squash, onion, and mushrooms in a large nonstick pan with olive oil.
2. Cook over medium to medium-high heat for about 7 minutes, or until the vegetables are just soft.
3. Take the vegetables out of the pan.
4. Put one tortilla in the same pan that has been sprayed with cooking spray. Evenly distribute
5. 1/4 cup of cheese over the tortilla, then cover the cheese with 3/4 cup of the vegetable mixture.
6. After adding an additional 1/8 cup of cheese to the veggies, cover them with a second tortilla.

Ingredients

- Six whole wheat tortillas (9 inches)
- a quarter cup of shredded low-fat sharp Cheese cheddar

Direction

7. Cook for 2 to 3 minutes on each side, or until golden on both sides.
8. Take the quesadilla out of the pan and continue with the rest of the ingredients.
9. Using a pizza cutter, cut each tortilla into eight triangles. Warm up the food.

FRUITY CURRY CHICKEN SALAD

A delicious and nutritious chicken salad with a fruity touch that tastes excellent in a honey

Pita or on a croissant.

Prep   **Cook**   **Serves**

45 Minutes   45 Minutes   8

Ingredients

- 4 cooked and chopped skinless, boneless chicken breast halves
- One chopped celery stalk
- four chopped green onions
- One chopped, peeled, and cored Golden Delicious apple
- Half a cup golden raisins
- ⅓ cup halved green grapes without seeds
- Chopped toasted pecans, ½ cup
- 1 tsp finely ground black pepper
- One-half teaspoon of curry powder
- ¾ cup of mild mayo

Direction

1. The chicken, celery, onion, apple, raisins, grapes, nuts, pepper, curry powder, and mayonnaise should all be combined in a big bowl.
2. Combine everything. Present!

COBB SALAD

Some of my favorite components in this Cobb salad are avocado, tomatoes, blue cheese, chicken, and egg.

Nutrition Facts

Calories – 525   Carbs – 40g

Fat – 10g   Protein – 32g

Prep   **Cook**   **Serves**
20 Minutes   10 Minutes   6

Ingredients

- 6 bacon pieces
- three eggs
- One head of shredded iceberg lettuce
- Three cups cooked and chopped chicken meat
- Two sliced and seeded tomatoes
- ¾ cup of shredded blue cheese
- three chopped green onions
- One chopped, pitted, and peeled avocado
- One 8-oz bottle of ranch-style salad dressing

Direction

1. Add the eggs to a saucepan, fill it all the way with cold water, bring to a boil, cover, and turn off the heat. Let eggs remain for ten to twelve minutes, then remove and cut, cool.

2. Place the bacon in a big, deep skillet and fry while the eggs cook. Simmer on medium-high heat for 7 to 10 minutes, or until uniformly browned. Shake well, crumble, and reserve.

3. Arrange the shredded lettuce on separate plates. Arrange bacon, eggs, chicken, tomatoes, green onions, blue cheese, and avocado in rows on top.

4. Pour dressing over.

BAKED SPLIT CHICKEN BREAST

This recipe for roasted chicken breasts is really simple, yet it appears like you spent hours in the kitchen, even if you hardly touched the stove!

Prep   **Cook**   **Serves**
10 Minutes   1 hr 30 min   2

Ingredients

- 2 big skin-and-bone-in chicken breast halves
- Half a cup of extra virgin olive oil.
- ½ teaspoon finely minced garlic
- A tsp of fine sea salt
- A tsp of finely ground black pepper
- One-half tsp of dried rosemary
- One-half teaspoon of dried basil

Direction

1. Gather all the ingredients.
2. Chicken breasts should be rubbed with garlic and olive oil and seasoned with salt, black pepper, rosemary, and basil. Chicken should be arranged in a big baking dish.
3. For at least 45 minutes, refrigerate. Meanwhile, heat the oven to 190 degrees Celsius, or 375 degrees Fahrenheit.
4. Bake the chicken for 45 to 60 minutes, or until the meat is no longer pink at the bone and the juices run clear, in a preheated oven. When the thickest portion of the breast meat is inserted, an instant-read thermometer should read 165 degrees Fahrenheit (75 degrees Celsius).
5. Enjoy while hot!

DINNER RECIPES

ASPARAGUS WITH SLICED ALMONDS AND PARMESAN CHEESE

This easy recipe transforms boring asparagus into a side dish that will please any man in your life! Serve alongside turkey meatballs or grilled fish.

Nutrition Facts

Calories – 178   Carbs – 7g

Fat – 14g   Protein – 8g

Prep   **Cook**   **Serves**

2 Minutes   12 Minutes   4

Ingredients

- Two tsp butter
- One pound of trimmed bottom asparagus
- ⅓ cup almonds, sliced
- One-half cup Parmesan cheese

Direction

1. In a big skillet set over medium-high heat, melt butter.
2. Add the asparagus and simmer for about 3 minutes while stirring.
3. Add the almonds and parmesan, then simmer for 3 to minutes, or until the cheese starts to color slightly.

EASY SHRIMP VEGETABLE STIR FRY

A simple and well-liked dinner is sweet caramelized shrimp stir-fried with vegetables on top of a fluffy bed of brown rice!

Nutrition Facts

Calories – 317   Carbs – 43g

Fat – 6g   Protein – 24g

Prep   **Cook**   **Serves**
20 Minutes   15 Minutes   6

Ingredients

- Two cups of quick brown rice
- 1/4 cup of water
- Six tsp soy sauce
- Six tsp water
- Half a cup of honey
- Cider vinegar, two tablespoons
- Two tsp cornstarch
- Two tsp olive oil
- Two chopped garlic cloves
- Two cups florets of broccoli
- One cup of tiny carrots

Direction

1. In a bowl that is safe to use in the microwave, mix rice and water.
2. Place a cover on and cook on high for about 8 minutes, or until the water is completely absorbed. Using a fork, fluff, cover, and set aside.
3. In a small bowl, whisk together soy sauce, water, honey, cider vinegar, and cornstarch; leave aside.
4. The olive oil should be warmed over medium heat in a nonstick skillet.
5. Garlic is added and cooked for ten seconds.
6. Add the broccoli, carrots, onion, and black pepper.

Ingredients

- One little white onion, finely sliced
- One-half teaspoon of black pepper
- One cup of freshly sliced mushrooms
- A pound and a half of raw medium shrimp, deveined and skinned

Direction

7. Cook and stir for approximately five minutes, or until the broccoli and carrots are soft.
8. Add the mushrooms and stir-fry for two minutes.
9. After taking the veggies out of the skillet, set them aside.
10. Place the skillet back on the burner and add the sauce mixture. Let it cook for a minute.
11. When the meat becomes opaque and the sauce thickens, add the shrimp and stir until they become a bright pink on the exterior, which should take about three minutes.
12. After adding the veggies to the pan, serve them over brown rice.

CHICKEN BROCCOLI RICE SKILLET

This pan of chicken, broccoli, and rice serves as a complete meal—entrée, vegetable, and rice—and is garnished with cheese. It is essentially a casserole that keeps the kitchen cool. On weeknights, it's a fantastic option for families.

Nutrition Facts

Calories – 512   Carbs – 21g

Fat – 27g   Protein – 45g

Prep   **Cook**   **Serves**
15 Minutes   38 Minutes   5

Ingredients

- One spoonful of butter
- One little onion, chopped
- One-pound chicken breast, skinless and boneless
- 1/4 cup optional orzo
- One box (6.3 ounces) of herb and garlic rice mix
- One and a quarter cups of chicken broth half a cup of milk

Direction

1. In a big, nonstick skillet set over medium heat, melt butter.
2. Cook and stir onions for about five minutes, or until they are tender and translucent.
3. Chop the chicken breast into small pieces in the interim.
4. Add the chicken to the skillet and cook, stirring, for about 5 minutes, or until browned. Add rice and orzo to skillet along with seasoning packet.
5. Combine the cream of chicken soup, milk, oregano, and garlic in a medium-sized bowl and transfer the mixture into the skillet. Mix well and add broccoli florets

Ingredients

Direction

6. Turn down the heat to low, cover, and simmer for about 25 minutes, or until the rice and orzo are bite-sized and the liquid has been absorbed.
7. After turning on the broiler, place a rack six inches below the heating element in the oven.
8. After scattering cheese over the skillet, broil for three minutes, or until the cheese is melted and golden.
9. Serve right away.

VEGETARIAN REFRIED BEANS

This is a spicy turkey chili made with four kinds of beans, salsa, chili powder, and loads of cumin.

Prep   **Cook**   **Serves**
15 Minutes   *1 hr 30 mins*   12

Ingredients

- 3 canned diced tomatoes with green chili peppers (15 ounces)
- Two fifteen-ounce cans of chili beans with a hot sauce
- One 16-oz jar of hot salsa
- One fifteen-ounce can of kidney beans, dark red
- One fifteen-ounce container of mild red kidney beans
- Two little onions, finely sliced
- Six smashed garlic cloves
- Two tsp of chili powder
- Two tablespoons of crushed red pepper

Direction

1. In a large soup pot, combine chopped tomatoes, green chiles, chili beans, salsa, black beans, dark and light red kidney beans, onions, garlic, cumin, black pepper, chili powder, and taco seasoning mix.

2. After reaching a boil, reduce the heat and place a lid on the pot.

3. Simmer the soup for about20 minutes, or until the onions are translucent and the soup is well heated.

4. 20 minutes, or until the onions are translucent and the soup is well heated.

Ingredients

Direction

5. Turn the heat up to medium-high and prepare a large skillet.

6. For about ten minutes, cook and mix the ground turkey in the heated skillet until it is browned and crumbly.

7. Then, drain and discard the fat. Mix the turkey crumbles into the chili.

8. Simmer the chili for one hour or until the flavors have melded, covered pot.

TOFU AND VEGGIES IN PEANUT

A simple and quick dinner of tofu and veggies with a delicious peanut butter sauce. A family favorite.

Prep   **Cook**   **Serves**

10 Minutes   10 Minutes   4

Ingredients

- One tablespoon of peanut oil
- One pound of diced firm tofu
- One small head of chopped broccoli
- One little red bell pepper, cut
- Five fresh, sliced mushrooms
- Half a cup of peanut butter. Half a cup of heated water
- Two tsp of vinegar
- Two tsp soy sauce
- A quarter of a cup molasses

Direction

1. Over medium-high heat, warm the oil in a large skillet or wok.
2. For five minutes, sauté the tofu, broccoli, bell pepper, and mushrooms.
3. In a small bowl, mix together peanut butter, boiling water, vinegar, soy sauce, molasses, and cayenne pepper.
4. Drizzle over the tofu and veggies. Simmer for 3 to 5 minutes, or until veggies are crisp-tender.

ZUCCHINI NOODLES SHRIMP

Although we adore shrimp scampi, we've made the decision to limit our intake of high-carb foods. This is the ideal resolution! I will be switching from pasta to vegetable noodles on a regular basis from now on!

Nutrition Facts

Calories – 161   Carbs – 87g

Fat – 25g   Protein – 9g

Prep
30 Minutes

Cook
15 Minutes

Serves
4

Ingredients

- 1 ½ pounds zucchini
- ¼ cup unsalted butter
- 2 tablespoons olive oil
- 1 shallot, minced
- 2 cloves garlic, minced
- ½ cup white wine
- ½ lemon, juiced
- 1 pound large shrimp, peeled and deveined
- salt and ground black pepper to taste

Direction

1. Use a julienne peeler or spiralizer to make zucchini noodles.
2. In a big skillet set over medium-high heat, melt butter.
3. Add a drizzle of olive oil. Add shallot; cook and stir for 4 to 5 minutes, or until tender.
4. Add the minced garlic and sauté for 2 minutes, or until golden.
5. Add the wine and lemon juice, and heat for about 3 minutes, or until the sauce has reduced by almost half.
6. Add the shrimp, black pepper, and salt. Cook for 2 to 3 minutes, or until shrimp turn pink.
7. The shrimp should be put on a serving plate.

Ingredients

- 2 tablespoons chopped fresh parsley, or to taste
- 2 tablespoons grated Parmesan cheese, or to taste (Optional)

Direction

1. Add the zucchini noodles to the skillet and stir.
2. Put some salt and black pepper over it. Cook for 4 to 6 minutes, or until noodles are soft.
3. Put the shrimp back in the skillet. Before serving, stir in the Parmesan cheese and parsley.

BAKED EGGPLANT PARMESAN

Baked eggplant Parmesan is a filling dish with Italian influences that consists of bread-crusted eggplant pieces baked with Parmesan cheese in between layers of tomato sauce and more cheese!

Nutrition Facts

Calories – 474   Carbs – 44g

Fat – 20g   Protein – 30g

Prep   **Cook**   **Serves**
20 Minutes   3hr 45 Minutes   6

Ingredients

- Peel and cut into 1/2-inch slices two eggplants.
- 1/4 cup salt, or more if necessary
- 1 cup bread crumbs in the Italian style
- Grated Parmesan cheese, ¼ cup
- Two beaten eggs
- One 28-oz jar of spaghetti sauce with tomatoes and garlic
- Grated Parmesan cheese, ¼ cup

Direction

1. After placing the eggplant slices in a colander, salt each slice on both sides. Let it settle for a minimum of three hours. Using paper towels, remove any surplus moisture from the eggplant slices.
2. Set the oven temperature to 175 degrees Celsius, or 350 degrees Fahrenheit. Grease a baking sheet.
3. In a small bowl, combine bread crumbs and 1/4 cup Parmesan cheese. In a different shallow bowl, beat eggs.
4. Place slices of eggplant in beaten egg. Raise the egg so that any extra falls back into the bowl.

Ingredients

- One package (16 ounces) of shredded mozzarella cheese, or more as required
- One-half teaspoon of dried basil

Cook's Note

There will be a lot of fresh taste added if you add fresh basil leaves in one of the layers. If you would like, you can also add fresh basil and garlic to the sauce. I like to add five to ten freshly picked basil leaves and two to four cloves of fresh garlic.

Direction

1. Place the breaded eggplant slices in a single layer on the baking sheet that has been prepared after pressing them into bread crumbs to coat both sides.

2. Bake for about five minutes on each side in a preheated oven, or until nicely browned and crisp.

3. Lay a layer of pasta sauce on the bottom and a layer of eggplant slices on top of it in a 9 x 13-inch casserole dish.

4. Add around one tablespoon of the leftover Parmesan and one-third of the mozzarella cheese.

5. Continue layering the remaining ingredients, then finish with a layer of cheese.

6. Add a few basil leaves.

7. Bake for about 35 minutes, or until the cheese is bubbling and golden brown, in a preheated oven.

LENTIL SOUP WITH SPINACH

This is a tasty and simple lentil soup. Add any extra vegetables you enjoy, even though the recipe only asks for spinach, potatoes, and carrots.

Prep
15 Minutes

Cook
1 hr 5 Minutes

Serves
12

Ingredients

- Four bacon slices, diced
- One cup of carrots, shredded
- One large onion, finely sliced
- One tsp olive oil
- Six cups of chicken stock
- Three cups of water
- One cup salsa
- Sixteen ounces of washed dried lentils
- One bay leaf
- One teaspoon of cumin powder

Direction

1. Place the bacon into a large skillet or Dutch oven and cook over medium-high heat until uniformly browned, about 10 minutes, rotating periodically.
2. After around five minutes, stir in the carrot, onion, and olive oil and simmer until soft.
3. Pour chicken stock, water, and salsa over the bacon mixture; stir in lentils, cumin, bay leaf, rosemary, salt, and pepper.
4. Over high heat, bring to a boil; then, lower the heat to a simmer, cover, and cook for 40 to 50 minutes, or until the lentils are soft..

Ingredients

- One tsp of dehydrated rosemary
- Spice up with black pepper and salt to taste.
- One 10-oz box of fresh spinach, ripped
- One cup of diced potatoes

Direction

5. Add the spinach and potatoes, and simmer for an additional 10 to 15 minutes, or until the spinach has wilted and the potatoes are tender.

This spicy turkey chili is made with four kinds of beans, salsa, chili powder, and loads of Cumin.

Nutrition Facts	
Calories – 319	Carbs – 41g
Fat – 9g	Protein – 10g

Prep
15 Minutes

Cook
1 hr. 30 minute

Serves
12

Ingredients

- 3 canned diced tomatoes with green chili peppers (15 ounces)
- Two fifteen-ounce cans of chili beans with a hot sauce
- One 16-oz jar of hot salsa
- One fifteen-ounce can of kidney beans, dark red
- One fifteen-ounce container of mild red kidney beans

Direction

1. In a large soup pot, combine chopped tomatoes, green chiles, chili beans, salsa, black beans, dark and light red kidney beans, onions, garlic, cumin, black pepper, chili powder, and taco seasoning mix.
2. Bring to a boil, then lower the heat and cover the pot.
3. Simmer for about 20 minutes, or until soup is heated through and onions are transparent.
4. A big skillet should be heated at medium-high heat. For about ten minutes, cook and mix the ground turkey in the heated

Ingredients

- One fifteen-ounce can of spiced black beans
- two little onions, finely sliced
- six smashed garlic cloves
- two tsp of chili powder
- Two tablespoons of crushed red pepper
- Two teaspoons of black pepper, ground coarsely
- two tsp finely ground cumin
- One package (1.25 ounces) of taco seasoning mix
- One tsp of hot sauce
- Two pounds of turkey meat

Direction

1. For about ten minutes, cook and mix the ground turkey in the heated skillet until it is browned and crumbly.
2. Then, drain and discard the fat. Mix the turkey crumbles into the chili.
3. Simmer the chili for one hour or until the flavors have melded, covered pot.

ROASTED BRUSSELS WITH SPROUT

Roasting Brussels sprouts is excellent for weekday dinners and very easy to create

Nutrition Facts

Calories – 319   Carbs – 41g

Fat – 9g   Protein – 10g

Prep   **Cook**   **Serves**

10 Minutes   30 minutes   6

Ingredients

- One entire pound of Brussels sprouts
- Four bacon slices, sliced into half-inch pieces
- Half a teaspoon of salt
- One-half teaspoon of newly ground black pepper
- Half a cup of extra virgin olive oil.
- Three teaspoons of pure maple syrup

Direction

1. Compile every component. Set the oven's temperature to 400°F, or 200°C. Use aluminum foil to line a baking sheet with a rim.
2. Cut large Brussels sprouts in half and trim the ends. Move to a large bowl.
3. Toss in bacon, pepper, and salt with the Brussels sprouts. After drizzling the sprouts with maple syrup and olive oil, toss them until well covered.
4. Spread out in a single layer on the baking sheet that has been ready.
5. Roast for 20 to 30 minutes, stirring halfway through, or until bacon is crispy and Brussels sprouts are caramelized in the preheated oven.
6. Enjoy and warm up!

SNACKS RECIPES

GREEK YOGURT BREAKFAST PARFAIT

Savor this tasty, adaptable Greek yogurt parfait for dessert or as a snack for breakfast

Nutrition Facts

Calories – 264   Carbs – 26g

Fat – 14g   Protein – 9g

Prep   **Cook**   **Serves**
15 Minutes   10 Minutes   2

Ingredients

- Half a cup of fresh blueberries
- ½ cup of freshly cut strawberries
- One tsp of white sugar, if desired
- Half a cup of granola, or as desired
- One 6-oz carton of vanilla Greek yogurt without fat
- One tsp lemon zest

Direction

1. Put the strawberries and blueberries in a small bowl.
2. Dredge in sugar and toss to coat the berries.
3. Put two teaspoons of granola into each of the two parfait glasses.
4. Top with 2 tablespoons of yogurt and 1/2 teaspoon of lemon zest.
5. Add a third of the berries on top. Once the parfait glasses are full, continue layering.

APPLE SMOOTHIE

Greek yogurt, banana, almond butter, and warm pie spices make this a delicious way to start the day or brighten up the afternoon.

Prep   **Cook**   **Serves**
5 Minutes   0 Minutes   1

Ingredients

- 1 small frozen-peeled banana
- One large Fuji apple, peeled and cut
- 3/4 cup Greek yogurt, full milk
- 1/4 cup of apple juice, unsweetened
- Three tsp rolled oats
- One spoonful of butter made of almonds
- two tsp maple syrup, or more to taste
- One pinch of ground cinnamon
- One dash of ground nutmeg
- One pinch of ground cloves

Direction

1. In the cup of a high-speed blender, combine the banana, apple, yogurt, apple juice, oats, almond butter, maple syrup, cinnamon, nutmeg, and cloves; mix until smooth.

2. If you'd like, you can thin the smoothie with milk or make it thicker with ice.

PINA COLADA COTTAGE

When you're not in the mood for yogurt, this cottage cheese bowl can satisfy your cravings! It tastes great and is healthy!

Prep   **Cook**   **Serves**

10 Minutes   10 Minutes   1

Ingredients

- ½ cup cottage cheese with little fat
- ¼ cup of freshly cut pineapple
- One tablespoon of toasted, unsweetened coconut
- One tablespoon of macadamia nuts, finely chopped
- One tablespoon of granola

Direction

1. Cottage cheese should be put in a small bowl. On top, arrange the granola, pineapple, coconut, and macadamia nuts side by side.
2. Serve right away.

EASY ROASTED RED PEPPER

A tasty dip or spread, this roasted red pepper hummus is made simply in a food processor with chickpeas, lemon juice, and tahini.

Prep   **Cook**   **Serves**

15 Minutes   0 Minutes   4

Ingredients

- 1 (15-ounce) bag of drained chickpeas
- One-third cup tahini
- One-third cup of lemon juice
- two minced garlic cloves
- ½ cup of roasted peppers, red
- One-half teaspoon of dried basil
- Add pepper and salt to taste (Optional)

Direction

1. In the bowl of a food processor, combine chickpeas, tahini, lemon juice, and garlic; pulse to blend. Process the roasted peppers until they are finely minced, then add the basil.
2. Add pepper and salt for seasoning.
3. Hummus should be moved to a small bowl, covered, and chilled until it's time to serve.

Cook's Note:

Many grocery stores carry tahini, a paste formed from sesame seeds.

You may prepare this hummus recipe a day in advance. Before serving, remove from the refrigerator and let it come to room temperature.

BACON BALSAMIC DEVILED EGGS

Makes a great recipe using light mayonnaise and sugar alternative; no taste difference is noticeable.

Prep   **Cook**   **Serves**

30 Minutes   *35 Minutes*   24

Ingredients

- 24 deviled eggs
- Components
- Twelve big eggs
- Four bacon slices
- Half a cup of mayonnaise
- Minced red onion, ¼ cup
- Two tsp white sugar
- One-half tsp balsamic vinegar
- One-half tspn celery salt
- One-half teaspoon of newly ground black pepper
- ¼ cup of freshly chopped parsley

Direction

1. Arrange the eggs in a single layer in a big pot and add one inch of water to cover. After bringing the water to a boil while covering the saucepan, turn off the heat and let the eggs in the hot water for fifteen minutes. Empty. Cool eggs in the sink with cold running water. Cut in half lengthwise and peel. After separating the yolks and whites, transfer the yolks to a bowl.

2. Place the rounded side of the egg whites down on a serving dish.

3. In a large, deep skillet, fry bacon over medium-high heat, flipping regularly, until uniformly browned, about 10 minutes, while the eggs are cooking. Drain onto a tray lined with paper towels; chop.

4. With a fork, mash the yolks. Incorporate the mayonnaise, bacon, onion, sugar, vinegar, celery salt, and pepper; mix well. Into the egg whites, spoon mixture. Add parsley as a garnish.

HOMEMADE MIX NUT BUTTER

This smooth, healthier substitute for store-bought peanut butter is here. Since it's a blend of numerous kind of nuts, you can adjust the amounts to suit your tastes.

Nutrition Facts

Calories – 208 Carbs – 9g

Fat – 18g   Protein – 7g

Prep   **Cook**   **Serves**
15 Minutes   10 Minutes   16

Ingredients

- 1/4 cup uncooked walnuts
- One-half cup raw almonds
- One-third cup raw, shelled, unsalted pistachios
- Two tablespoons of granulated sucralose (Splenda-style sweetener)
- One tablespoon of honey
- One tablespoon of essence from vanilla
- Half a teaspoon of salt

Direction

1. Set the oven temperature to 175 degrees Celsius, or 350 degrees Fahrenheit. Arrange the pistachios, almonds, and walnuts on a baking sheet with a rim.

2. Bake the nuts for 10 to 15 minutes, or until they are fragrant and toasted, in a preheated oven.

3. While still hot, transfer to a food processor and process at high speed until crumbly and beginning to clump. Switch off the processor and use a spatula to scrape down the sides.

4. Process once more until a cream begins to form. Blend for a minute after adding sucralose, honey, vanilla extract, and salt.

Ingredients

- ⅓ cup powdered dark cocoa (Optional)
- Three tablespoons of powdered nonfat dry milk (optional)

Direction

5. Process for an additional minute after adding the cocoa powder and milk powder in turns.
6. Allow to cool fully. Move to a jar and store in the refrigerator.

Cook's Note:

If using cocoa powder, only use non-fat dry milk.

To make the spread chunkier, simply add chopped nuts.

STRAW BERRY AVOCADO SALAD

I use this dressing on a lot of other salads and have served it a lot; every time, someone asks for the recipe. Have fun!

Prep   **Cook**   **Serves**

15 Minutes   15 Minutes   2

Ingredients

- Two tsp of white sugar
- Two tsp olive oil
- four tsp honey
- One tablespoon of apple cider vinegar
- one tsp lemon juice
- two cups of shredded lettuce
- One avocado, cut, pitted, and peeled
- ten sliced strawberries
- ½ cup of pecans, chopped

Direction

1. Combine the sugar, lemon juice, vinegar, honey, and olive oil in a small bowl. Put aside.
2. Top a lovely bowl of salad greens with sliced avocado and strawberries.
3. Pour dressing over all of it, and then top with pecans.
4. Serve right away, or refrigerate for up to two hours before serving.

AIR FRYER CELERY FRIES

Delicious fries cooked in an air fryer with celery root and served hot with vegan mayonnaise

Prep   **Cook**   **Serves**
20 Minutes   28 Minutes   4

Ingredients

- ½ peeled and chopped celeriac (celery root), cut into 1/2-inch sticks
- three cups of water
- One tablespoon of lime juice
- Mayonnaise Sauce:
- One-third cup vegan mayo
- One tablespoon of mustard brown
- One teaspoon of horseradish powder
- One tablespoon of olive oil
- Spice up with a small teaspoon of salt and ground black pepper.

Direction

1. Place the root celery in a bowl. Add lime juice and water. Stir, then leave for twenty minutes.
2. Set the air fryer's temperature to 400°F, or 200°C.
3. Prepare the mayonnaise. Combine the horseradish powder, mustard, and vegan mayonnaise. Store in the refrigerator with a cover until needed.
4. After draining and drying, return the celery root sticks to a basin. Sprinkle salt and pepper on top of the fries and drizzle with oil. For an even coat, toss.
5. Fill the air fryer basket with celery root. Cook for about 10 minutes, checking the food for doneness halfway through. Fry for a further 8 minutes or until the fries are crisp and golden, shaking the basket occasionally.
6. Serve fries right away with a side of vegan mayo.

FRIED MOZALLERAL CHEESE STICKS

Making mozzarella sticks at home is quite simple. The inside is filled with melting, gooey cheese and the exterior is golden and crispy from deep-frying. Fry these for only a few minutes, and they taste very amazing! Give them a marinara sauce dip!

Nutrition Facts

Calories – 789 Carbs – 30g

Fat –67g   Protein – 19g

Prep   **Cook**   **Serves**

15 Minutes   10 Minutes   8

Ingredients

- Two big, beaten eggs
- Half a cup water
- 1/2 cup of seasoned Italian bread crumbs
- Half a teaspoon of salt with garlic
- ⅔ Cup flour for all purposes
- One-third cup cornstarch
- Two cups of frying oil, or more as needed
- One package (16 ounces) of mozzarella cheese

Direction

1. In a small bowl, whisk together eggs and water. In a medium-sized bowl, combine bread crumbs and garlic powder. In a third bowl, blend together flour and cornstarch.
2. In a big, heavy saucepan, heat oil to 365 degrees Fahrenheit (185 degrees Celsius).
3. A mozzarella stick should be floured and the excess shaken off. Dive into the mixture of eggs. Raise up so that any extra egg falls back into the bowl. Coat by pressing into bread crumbs. Spread the breaded mozzarella stick onto a wire rack or platter. Continue with the leftover mozzarella sticks.
4. Lower three to four mozzarella sticks into the heated oil using a spider spoon or a pair of tongs. Fry for about 30 seconds, or until golden brown. Take out of the heat and let dry on paper towels. Continue frying the leftover mozzarella sticks.
5. Enjoy and serve hot.

SZECHUAN EDAMAME

This quick and tasty soybean dish makes a great, high-protein snack that can easily take the place of potato chips. Warm up and serve. Note: The outer pod of this bean is not edible!

Nutrition Facts	
Calories – 233	Carbs – 10g
Fat – 23g	Protein – 14g

Prep **Cook** **Serves**
15 Minutes 4 hour 12

Ingredients

- 1 package (16 ounces) frozen edamame in the pod
- Two tsp sesame seeds
- Three teaspoons of white sugar
- Two tsp soy sauce
- Two tsp olive oil
- To taste, add up to 1 teaspoon of red pepper flakes.

Direction

1. Put the edamame pods and 1/4 cup water in a microwave-safe bowl. Place a cover on and cook on high for 4 to 6 minutes, or until soft. Empty.
2. Sesame seeds should be lightly toasted for about two minutes in a skillet over medium heat.
3. Stir in sugar, red pepper flakes, olive oil, and soy sauce. Simmer for about two minutes, or until soy sauce reduces and becomes somewhat thicker. Toss in the edamame and heat for an additional minute or two.
4. If preferred, you can use vegetable oil in place of the olive oil.
5. Simply leave off the red pepper flakes if you don't want them to be overly hot, or add more if you want a little more kick.

31 DAY MEAL PLAN

	BREAKFAST	LUNCH	DINNER
DAY 1	Summer Berry Parfait with Yogurt and Granola	Extreme Veggie Scrambled Eggs	Asparagus with Sliced Almonds and Parmesan Cheese
DAY 2	Overnight Buckwheat Oats	Overnight Buckwheat Oats	Fried Mozalleral Cheese Sticks
DAY 3	Chocolate-Banana-Peanut Butter Smoothie	Buddha Bowl	Chicken Broccoli Rice Skillet
DAY 4	Extreme Veggie Scrambled Eggs	Yummy Veggie Omelet	Spicy Turkey Bean Chili
DAY 5	Cucumber Cups with Dill Cream and Smoked Salmon	Chicken Salad Wraps	Tofu and Veggies in Peanut Sauce
DAY 6	Banana Pancakes	Chocolate Chip Cinnamon Cookies	Zucchini Noodle Shrimp Scampi
DAY 7	Curried Cashew, Pear, and Grape Salad	Farmer's Market Vegetarian Quesadillas	Baked Eggplant Parmesan

	BREAKFAST	LUNCH	DINNER
DAY 8	**Meatless Sweet Potato Burrito Bowl**	**Fruity Curry Chicken Salad**	**Lentil Soup with Spinach**
DAY 9	**Avocado Toast with Egg**	**Cobb Salad**	**Maple Roasted Brussels Sprouts**
DAY 10	**Cinnamon-Peach Cottage Cheese Pancakes**	**Baked Split Chicken Breast**	**Cauliflower Chicken Fried Rice**
DAY 11	**Easy Shrimp Vegetable Stir Fry**	**Apple Smoothie**	**Overnight Buckwheat Oats**
DAY 12	**Chicken Broccoli Rice Skillet**	**Pina Colada Cottage Cheese**	**Chocolate-Banana-Peanut Butter Smoothie**
DAY 13	**Spicy Turkey Bean Chili**	**Easy Roasted Red Pepper**	**Extreme Veggie Scrambled Eggs**
DAY 14	**Tofu and Veggies in Peanut Sauce**	**Bacon Balsamic Deviled Eggs**	**Cucumber Cups with Dill Cream and Smoked Salmon**

	BREAKFAST	LUNCH	DINNER
DAY 15	**Chicken Salad Wraps**	**Fruity Curry Chicken Salad**	**Bacon Balsamic Deviled Eggs**
DAY 16	**Chocolate Chip Cinnamon Cookies**	**Zucchini Noodle Shrimp Scampi**	**Homemade Mixed Nut Butter on Whole Grain Toast**
DAY 17	**Farmer's Market Vegetarian Quesadillas**	**Baked Eggplant Parmesan**	**Strawberry Avocado Salad**
DAY 18	**Fruity Curry Chicken Salad**	**Lentil Soup with Spinach**	**Air Fryer Celery Root Fries**
DAY 19	**Cobb Salad**	**Maple Roasted Brussels Sprouts**	**Fried Mozzarella Cheese Sticks**
DAY 20	**Baked Split Chicken Breast**	**Cauliflower Chicken Fried Rice**	**Szechuan Edamame (Soy Beans)**
DAY 21	**Zucchini Noodle Shrimp Scampi**	**Homemade Mixed Nut Butter on Whole Grain Toast**	**Banana Pancakes**

	BREAKFAST	**LUNCH**	**DINNER**
DAY 22	Baked Eggplant Parmesan	Strawberry Avocado Salad	Strawberry Avocado Salad
DAY 23	Lentil Soup with Spinach	Air Fryer Celery Root Fries	Farmer's Market Vegetarian Quesadillas
DAY 24	Asparagus with Sliced Almonds and Parmesan Cheese	Greek Yogurt Breakfast Parfait	Air Fryer Celery Root Fries
DAY 25	Maple Roasted Brussels Sprouts	Fried Mozzarella Cheese Sticks	Cinnamon-Peach Cottage Cheese Pancakes
DAY 26	Cauliflower Chicken Fried Rice	Szechuan Edamame (Soy Beans)	High-Protein Vegan Stir-Fry
DAY 27	Greek Yogurt Breakfast Parfait	Summer Berry Parfait with Yogurt and Granola	Avocado Toast with Egg
DAY 28	Greek Yogurt Breakfast Parfait	Chicken Salad Wraps	Baked Salmon with Roasted Vegetables

	BREAKFAST	LUNCH	DINNER
DAY 29	Banana Pancakes	Quinoa Salad with Chickpeas and Feta	Turkey Meatballs with Marinara Sauce and Zucchini Noodles
DAY 30	Avocado Toast with Egg	Lentil Soup with Spinach	Grilled Chicken Breast with Steamed Broccoli
DAY 31	Spinach and Feta Omelet	Greek Salad with Grilled Shrimp	Vegetable Stir-Fry with Tofu

CONCLUSION

As we reach the end of this journey through intermittent fasting for women over seventy, we must look back on what we have done and achieved. We explored the science behind intermittent fasting and how it can be used to improve our health, as well as how it can be incorporated into our daily lives. The different kinds of fasting were also considered and those that suit us best were identified. We also talked about the necessity of heeding our body's needs and making necessary changes.

But perhaps most importantly, we have seen firsthand the transformative power of intermittent fasting. We lost stubborn weight, reduced joint pain, and increased energy levels; hence improved overall health status. It has helped us get back in control of our bodies and our life context.

Moving forward therefore, let us continue embracing the principles of intermittent fasting which will become part of our lives permanently. Therefore let's maintain focus on our health and well-being while listening to what feels right for our bodies to support these aspirations. Thus a healthier life can be constructed by us for ourselves as well as the next generations.

Thanks so much for staying with me all along this way; I wish you luck as you keep absorbing yourself in the world of intermittent fasting to have a healthier life full of happiness